# PRAISE FOR XANET PAILET

As someone who's spent my career advocating for women's sexual pleasure, I deeply appreciate how Xanet Pailet brings that same lens to the complex dance of couples' intimacy. The Sex and Intimacy Repair Kit honors women's needs while guiding both partners back to connection, communication, and mutual pleasure. It's a compassionate and practical roadmap for couples who are ready to repair and reawaken their sex lives—together.

—Laurie Mintz, PhD, author of *Becoming Cliterate* and *A Tired Woman's Guide to Passionate Sex*

If you're in a sexless or unsatisfying relationship, Xanet Pailet can help you. Her book, *The Sex and Intimacy Repair Kit*, lets you 'eavesdrop' on real couples' coaching sessions from her intimacy retreats as she guides them to express their needs, face their fears, and create a new path toward intimacy. You'll learn a lot about yourself as you enter Pailet's world.

—Joan Price, best-selling author of *Naked at Our Age: Talking Out Loud About Senior Sex*

There are few books that enter the sacred space between two people and manage to tell the truth with this much tenderness. *The Sex & Intimacy Repair Kit* is one of them.

As someone who has spent decades inside the emotional landscapes of couples, I've seen how fragile the bond between partners can feel when the tools for repair are missing. What Xanet Pailet offers here is not a list of techniques or scripts to follow, but an invitation to understand how love actually works when it is tested. This book teaches what most of us were never taught: how to rebuild safety where it was lost, how to hear without defending, how to stay open when shame tells us to close.

Every page is infused with compassion for the real struggles of intimacy. It honors the complexity of sex, of desire, of fear, of longing. Xanet brings to this work a rare combination of psychological precision and soulful wisdom. She reminds us that the path to deeper connection isn't found through performance or perfection, but through presence, the kind that can sit in truth, in discomfort, and still choose closeness.

This book is more than a guide; it's a mirror. It reflects the parts of us that still hope to be met, still want to trust, still want to love fully. Whether you are a therapist, a couple in crisis, or someone quietly yearning for more depth in your relationship, these pages will move you.

If you read slowly, if you practice what she invites you to try, this book will not just change your relationship; it will change your nervous system's understanding of safety, care, and love itself.

—Derek Hart, Couples Counselor, Educator, and Founder of *Attachment University*

In the Sex and Intimacy Repair Kit, Xanet has done an excellent job distilling an array of knowledge gathered from psychology, sexology, trauma healing, and self-help to make it accessible and helpful to any couple wanting to improve their relationship. Her personal experiences, client stories, and practical exercises offer illustrative insights and tools to create transformation and healing. I highly recommend this book to any couple wishing to feel more love and fulfillment in their sexual and emotional connection.

—Danielle Harel, PhD, Cofounder of Somatica Institute and author of *Coming Together* and *Making Love Real*

I love this book. It is the antidote to disconnection and mediocre sex in long-term committed relationships. This is an essential book that can help couples avoid the bad habits that destroy intimacy. It is full of relatable stories, advice, and exercises that all couples need to keep their passion and love alive. If your goal is to have a great relationship that lasts, you definitely must read this wonderful and eminently useful book.

—Lesli Dores, LMFT, marriage coach and best-selling author of *Blueprint for a Lasting Marriage* and *The Hero Husband Project*

The Sex and Intimacy Repair Kit is a brave, compassionate, and deeply practical guide for anyone longing for more emotional honesty and connection in their relationships. The chapter on vulnerability struck me in particular, offering a clear and humanizing exploration of how shame, emotional suppression, and early conditioning shape our capacity for intimacy. In my work with survivors of sexual abuse, I see every day how courageously people long to be known and loved, yet often feel blocked by the very patterns this book helps unravel. With its blend of personal story, science, and real-world tools, this book offers a path toward emotional safety, genuine closeness, and the kind of healing that makes intimacy possible again.

—Rachel Grant, MA, author of *Beyond Surviving: The Final Stage in Recovery from Sexual Abuse*

The Sex & Intimacy Repair Kit is the playbook for couples who refuse to live like 'roommates with rings,' wondering where the spark went. Xanet Pailet serves up real talk—and real tools—with bold, unfiltered stories that tear down walls and rebuild what actually matters: desire, emotional connection, and that *"meet me in the bedroom... now"* fire. This isn't theories and textbook fluff. This is action; this is courage. This is for couples who *know* they're meant for more and are ready to *level up*—even if stress, resentment, and years of avoiding the hard conversations have taken over between the sheets.

—L. Scott Ferguson, host of the *Time to Shine Today* podcast

*The Sex and Intimacy Repair Kit* is a gift to couples who are struggling and want to feel closer—emotionally, sexually, and in every way that truly matters. As a teacher who trains sex and relationship coaches in the Somatica Method, I know how powerful highly competent support can be—and how hard it is for many couples to access that level of care. Xanet has created something special: a book that brings the heart and skills of a highly trained sex and relationship professional directly into your home.

This book is filled with practical, step-by-step exercises that gently guide partners into deeper communication, greater understanding, and more authentic intimacy. Xanet draws from multiple modalities, including the Somatica Method, making it easy for couples to discover what resonates most and what actually works for them. Many of the practices in this book are similar to the ones I use with couples in my own practice.

What I especially love is how open and self-revealing Xanet is about her own journey. Her honesty helps normalize so much of what couples struggle with, helping readers release shame, break through loneliness, and feel more hopeful. This isn't just a practical how-to book—it's also an invitation to grow, heal, and reconnect in ways that can create a lifetime of passionate intimacy.

—Kai Wu, Sex and Relationship Coach and faculty member at the Somatica Institute

# THE SEX AND INTIMACY REPAIR KIT

## HOW TO ENHANCE COMMUNICATION AND CREATE A LIFETIME OF PASSIONATE INTIMACY

XANET PAILET

Published by Books That Save Lives, an imprint of Jim Dandy Publishing, LLC

Cover Design: Carmen Fortunato



Published by BTSL/Jim Dandy Publishing
6252 Peach Avenue
Van Nuys, CA 91411
info@jimdandypublishing.com

For bulk orders, special quantities, course adoptions, and corporate sales, please email info@jimdandypublishing.com

ISBN: (print) 978-1963667417, (ebook) 978-1963667721

BISAC: FAM029000, SEL034000

# CONTENTS

**A Note About Words Used in This Book:**

One of the challenges couples often face in communicating about sex is discomfort with talking about—and even naming—their genitals. This discomfort is a reflection of the shame-based sexual culture many of us were raised in. Because my mission is to help normalize and heal sexual shame, you will find that I use a range of words for sexual body parts throughout this book.

Sometimes the language is anatomically correct (such as vulva, vagina, penis, or testicles), and sometimes it reflects the more colloquial or erotic language people naturally use, including words like pussy or cock. This choice is intentional and meant to reflect real-world conversations, reduce fear around sexual language, and invite greater ease, honesty, and self-acceptance in how we talk about sex.

*For every couple desiring days filled with tenderness and understanding and nights alive with passion and pleasure.*

# FOREWORD

Every great relationship faces challenges. Every couple, no matter how strong, hits moments where connection fades, intimacy slips away, and they start feeling more like teammates than lovers. And far too many couples quietly accept this, believing there's no path back to passion, no roadmap to reconnection.

I'm here to tell you: *That is absolutely not true.* And this book is the proof.

*The Sex and Intimacy Repair Kit* by Xanet Pailet is more than just a book—it's a *playbook* for transforming your relationship from the inside out. Xanet gives you the tools, the strategies, and the mindset shifts you need to rebuild emotional safety, revive intimacy, and reignite the passion you thought was gone for good.

What I love about Xanet's work is that she doesn't shy away from the truth: Intimacy isn't just about sex. It's about connection, trust, communication, vulnerability, and the willingness to show up—fully and courageously—for your partner. She breaks down emotional intimacy, sexual intimacy, and the foundations of connection in a way that empowers you to take action immediately.

And let me tell you, when Xanet shares her personal story and why she's devoted her life to this work, it hits hard. I respected her before —I admired her after. Her transparency helps you lean in, learn more deeply, and believe in what's possible for your own relationship.

Her section on emotional intimacy is a masterclass. She teaches you how to create emotional safety—the kind of safety that allows love, passion, and connection to thrive. Because when your partner feels supported, valued, and truly seen, that's when intimacy skyrockets.

And the way she talks about sexual intimacy is powerful. Sex isn't about performing. It's not about pressure or expectations. It's about creating a space where two people can explore, connect, and experience pleasure without fear or judgment. That shift alone can transform your entire relationship.

This isn't theory. This is *results-driven coaching* in book form.

If you're willing to show up, lean in, and do the work, this book can absolutely change your relationship—and your life. I've read a lot of books on relationships and personal growth, and this one stands out because it's honest, it's practical, and it's written with real heart.

So here's my message to you:

If you're ready to bring back the spark...

If you're ready to communicate in a deeper way...

If you're ready to experience intimacy that's passionate, connected, and fulfilling...

*You are holding the right book in your hands.*

I give my strongest recommendation to *The Sex and Intimacy Repair Kit* and to the powerful work Xanet Pailet is offering couples everywhere. This book is your invitation to rebuild, reignite, and rise together.

Let's get to work.

—Marques Ogden, host of *Get Authentic with Marques Ogden* (Top 1% Podcast) and IOFP Top Inspirational Business Mentor of the Year 2024-2025

# INTRODUCTION BY THE AUTHOR

In 2018, I published my first best-selling book, *Living an Orgasmic Life: Heal Yourself and Awaken Your Pleasure.* My Orgasmic Life book both chronicled the journey of my own sexual healing and awakening and guided thousands of women to reclaim their own sexuality and desire. I was humbled by the response, and by the hundreds of emails I received from women and some men thanking me for helping to transform their sex life. I've also had the honor to personally coach hundreds of clients through their own journeys of awakening, helping them to heal sexual shame, abuse, and trauma.

As my experience grew, it became increasingly evident that my next focus was to work with couples who, like me, had been living in sexless marriages and were often on the brink of divorce. This part of my practice began with some couples' workshops where I introduced some of the concepts of connection and intimacy. The positive feedback I received from these events encouraged me to delve deeper into understanding couple relationship dynamics and ultimately creating a comprehensive program specifically geared towards couples, using an interactive, experiential approach.

For the past five years, I have poured my heart and soul into facilitating private and group Passionate Intimacy Retreats for couples. Through these powerful and transformative experiences, I have witnessed countless marriages being saved, relationships healed from infidelity and other deep wounds, and unhealthy patterns being broken. The atmosphere at my retreats is one of vulnerability, trust, curiosity, and growth. It's a safe haven where couples can let go of their masks and truly connect with each other on a deeper level. It brings me immense joy to see the incredible transformations that take place during these retreats and the lasting impact these experiences have on the couples' lives.

But unfortunately, there are only so many weekends in a year, and I know there are so many more couples who can benefit from this work. That's why I decided to write this book; I wanted to expand my reach and share these transformative tools and insights with a wider audience. Within these pages, you'll find the essence of what I've learned through years of working intimately with couples distilled into practical exercises, powerful mindset shifts, and heartfelt wisdom.

As I sat down to write, I found myself transported back to all the powerful moments I've witnessed over the years: the tears of relief as partners finally felt truly seen and heard; the laughter that spontaneously burst forth as playfulness was rekindled; the tender embraces as walls came down and hearts opened.

Before you dive in, take a moment to discover your own unique *Intimacy Equation*—the personal blend of heart, body, and energy that shapes how you love and connect. You'll learn how you naturally build closeness, when you get out of sync, and how to bring passion and harmony back into your relationship.

Take the free quiz at https://www.howtoimprovemylovelife.com

As you embark on this journey through the book, I invite you to approach it with an open heart and mind. Although some of the exercises may push you out of your comfort zone, remember that growth often happens at the edges of our comfort. Be patient with yourself and your partner as you navigate this path together.

Each chapter focuses on a different aspect of passionate intimacy—from reigniting the spark of desire to healing past hurts—and discovering new depths of emotional and physical connection.

I've included real stories from couples I've worked with (their names have been changed for privacy, of course) sharing their struggles and breakthroughs to inspire and encourage you. You'll also find practical exercises and prompts to help you apply the concepts to your own relationship. Since I primarily work with heterosexual couples, I'm writing this book through a heteronormative lens, which is also reflected in most of the case studies.  If you are a queer couple, you will find that the concepts and exercises will be relatable and useful in your intimate relationship. However, I do not delve into the nuances of queer sexuality since that is not my area of expertise.

My hope is that this book will serve as a guide and companion on your journey to deeper intimacy and connection. Whether you're in a long-term relationship looking to reignite the spark, newly committed and wanting to build a strong foundation, or somewhere in between, there's something here for you.

As you read, you might find yourself nodding in recognition, tearing up with emotion, or even feeling a bit uncomfortable at times. That's all part of the process. Growth and transformation often involve facing our fears and insecurities head-on. But I promise you, the rewards are worth it.

I encourage you to take your time with this book: Don't rush through it. Pause to reflect, discuss with your partner, and most importantly, put the exercises into practice. The real magic happens when you apply these principles in your daily life.

The path to passionate intimacy isn't always smooth. There will be challenges, moments of vulnerability, and perhaps even some tears along the way. Deeper connection, the joy of being truly seen and accepted, the thrill of continual discovery with your partner—these are the gifts that await you on the other side of this journey.

# PART ONE
# UNDERSTANDING THE FOUNDATION OF INTIMACY

In this section of the book, we explore the foundations of intimacy, starting with my own personal journey, which sets the stage for why I'm so passionate about this work. We examine the blocks to intimacy that couples experience and the three stages of sexual relationships, as well as learning some important tools, such as active and empathetic listening, that begin to create the emotional safety necessary for intimacy. Finally, we delve deeply into your intimacy blueprint, uncovering how childhood wounds and experiences shape our ability to form healthy adult relationships.

# I

# FROM HEALTHCARE LAWYER TO SEX AND INTIMACY COACH

If you had told me years ago that I'd be a sex and intimacy coach today, I probably would have laughed (or blushed) and said, "Not a chance." My journey here has been anything but straightforward, and honestly, the relationship I had with my body and my sexuality for most of my life was far from easy. This wasn't something that came naturally, nor was it a path that was preordained.

Those of you who've read my first book, *Living an Orgasmic Life: Heal Yourself and Awaken Your Pleasure*, have seen the nitty-gritty details of my sexual healing and awakening. That book was my deep dive into the wounds I had to heal and the work I had to do to find pleasure and joy in my own skin. But for those of you just meeting me here, let me give you the Cliff Notes version of how I got to this point— it's a bit of a ride.

It all started in first grade, of all places. I was just a curious kid, playing doctor with my best friend Josephine. We were innocent, experimenting with the kind of curiosity that's completely natural at that age. But when the grown-ups got involved, it became something much bigger.

My mom was called, Josephine and I were banned from having playdates, and just like that, our friendship was torn apart. To make matters worse, her family moved away that summer. For years, I carried this crushing guilt, convinced I was responsible for my best friend disappearing from my life. That was the first time shame around sex planted itself in my world, and it stuck around for decades.

Then there was Lucky. He was our high-strung little Yorkshire terrier, yappy and hyper, and honestly, not my favorite companion. But Lucky had other plans. One day, out of the blue, he took an interest in licking my underwear. I remember feeling something unexpected—a kind of pleasure I hadn't experienced before. And if I'm being completely honest, Lucky probably gave me my first orgasm.

Now, you might be thinking this would have been a breakthrough moment—some kind of doorway to sexual freedom and body positivity, right? Wrong. It was more like a door slamming shut, trapping me in a space filled with confusion and shame. My sexuality became something I didn't understand, and instead of feeling free, I felt even more disconnected.

From that day on, anything having to do with sex and the female body, including menstruation, created a tremendous amount of fear, shame, and anxiety in me. The mere mention of these topics would send shivers down my spine and make my stomach churn. So it's no surprise that when I lost my virginity at age sixteen with my boyfriend Stephen, the pain was unbearable. After that experience, any kind of sexual intercourse or penetration was usually met with intense discomfort and tears. It was definitely not the ideal start to a healthy sex life.

To make matters worse, orgasms were completely elusive for me. Despite my curiosity and desire to explore my sexuality, the physical and emotional barriers I faced made it difficult for me to engage in sexual relationships during college.

However, there was an ironic twist to all of this and a foreshadowing of my future path. Even though sex was largely off-limits for me, I found myself drawn to helping others in this area. In fact, I became a sexual peer counselor at my college, educating women about birth control options (the diaphragm was all the rage back then because getting a prescription for the pill was often more challenging), STDs, and pregnancy termination alternatives.

On the surface, it seemed like a great fit for me—using my knowledge and passion to assist others in navigating their own sexual health. But deep down, I couldn't help feeling envious of those who could freely enjoy their own sexuality while I struggled with mine.

It should come as no surprise that when my now-ex-husband and I met in my first year of law school, our sexual intimacy was far from euphoric. He was weighed down by the weight of a family tragedy, and I found myself struggling to connect with him physically.

My body was also beginning to give me signs—unspoken messages that I couldn't understand or articulate. Chronic bladder and vaginal infections plagued me, further distancing me from my own sexuality and physical self. It wasn't long before—at the ripe age of twenty-eight and after giving birth to our second child—I closed off completely, shutting the door on any physical intimacy. For over two decades, our marriage became devoid of any sexual connection or passion. It was like living in a loveless desert, with no oasis in sight.

My life was consumed by my job as an executive at various national health care organizations, taking care of my two boys, producing theater in New York City on the side, spending time with my girlfriends, and hitting the gym

I was the epitome of the high-achieving, type A personality—always busy, always productive, and always running from the emptiness I felt inside. On the surface, I had it all together: a successful career, beautiful children, and a comfortable life. But underneath, there was a void that no amount of professional success or motherly pride could fill.

It wasn't until I turned fifty that I finally reached a breaking point. The facade I had carefully constructed began to crumble, and I could no longer ignore the deep dissatisfaction and disconnection I felt. What was left of my marriage had disintegrated, my career felt increasingly hollow, and I was tired—bone-deep tired—of running from myself.

That's when I made the terrifying decision to leave my marriage and my career behind. It was like stepping off a cliff, not knowing if there would be solid ground beneath me or if I'd just keep falling.

I stepped out of my marriage and into the world of online dating, which was beyond terrifying, given my belief that I was a broken woman and would never find another partner since I hated sex. Even though I weighed a sleek 110 pounds, my body image was distorted. I saw myself as unattractive and undesirable. The thought of being intimate with someone new filled me with dread.

But life has a way of surprising you when you least expect it. Through online dating, I met a man who would become a catalyst for change in my life. He was patient, understanding, and most importantly, he introduced me to the world of Tantra or sacred sexuality.

Our first intimate encounter was nothing short of transformative. For the first time in my life, I experienced pleasure without pain. It was as if a switch had been flipped, illuminating a part of myself I had long kept in darkness.

At first, I was skeptical. Tantra seemed like some new-age mumbo jumbo, far removed from my practical, logical world of healthcare law. But as I began to explore Tantra, something inside me started to shift. For the first time in decades, I felt a glimmer of hope that maybe, just maybe, I could heal my relationship with my body and my sexuality.

My sexual healing and awakening journey was arduous. I landed in California, leaving behind my home, my grown children, and my friends on the East Coast. But I was determined to forge a new path on my own.

Over the next few years, I took a deep dive into sexuality. Through a variety of training programs, I was able to work through my shame around sex, the medical trauma I had experienced at the hands of urologists trying in vain to cure my bladder infections, and the lingering effects of my early experiences.

I immersed myself in countless workshops, retreats, and training programs focused on sexual healing. Each experience peeled back another layer of shame and trauma, revealing glimpses of the vibrant, sensual woman I had the potential to become.

It wasn't always easy. There were moments of profound discomfort, buckets of tears, and times when I wanted to run back to the safety of my old life. But something kept pushing me forward—a deep-seated desire to finally be free, to finally feel whole.

One particularly transformative experience came during a week-long retreat in the mountains. On the third day, we were guided through a partner exercise involving eye gazing and gentle touch. As I sat across from my partner, a kind-eyed stranger, I felt waves of emotion wash over me. Tears streamed down my face as I allowed myself to be truly seen, perhaps for the first time in my life. In that moment, I realized how much I had been hiding, not just from others, but from myself.

As I healed, I began to realize that my journey wasn't just for me. The skills and knowledge I was gaining could help others who were struggling with similar issues. I started to see how my background in healthcare and my personal journey, combined with my growing expertise in sexuality and intimacy, could create a unique and powerful new career for me.

It wasn't an easy transition—making the shift from being a high-powered healthcare executive to a sex and intimacy coach felt like stepping into an entirely different world. But with each client I met and each workshop I led, I felt more and more aligned with my true purpose.

As a lawyer with a thirst for knowledge, I eagerly enrolled in various sex and intimacy training programs. Over the course of several years, I dedicated myself to becoming an expert in this realm, earning certifications as a Somatica® sex and intimacy coach, a Tantra Educator, a holistic pelvic care practitioner for women, and a Sexological Body Worker. But my journey didn't stop there. More recently, I completed an intensive three-year trauma training program and am now also a certified Somatic Experiencing Practitioner. My passion for understanding and helping others navigate their sexual and intimate lives knows no bounds.

Over the course of my (hard for me to believe) fourteen-year career, I have worked with hundreds of clients, both men and women, helping them to heal their own traumas and wounds and create the intimate relationships they truly desire. It's been a journey of constant learning, growth, and profound transformation —not just for my clients, but for me as well. My work has also reached thousands of others through my best-selling book, *Living an Orgasmic Life: Heal Yourself and Awaken Your Pleasure.* I have received countless messages from readers expressing how my book has changed their lives, and reading them never fails to bring tears to my eyes.

But perhaps the most profound transformation has been my own. That scared, ashamed little girl who couldn't even say the word 'sex' without blushing has blossomed into a woman who not only embraces her sexuality but celebrates it. I've learned to love my body, to honor my desires, and to cultivate deep, meaningful connections with others.

Now, at 66, I feel more alive, more vibrant, and more in touch with my sexuality than I ever did in my twenties or thirties. I'm living proof that it's never too late to heal, to grow, to change.

It's been fourteen years since I finally began to heal my sexuality, but along the way, I've also grown personally in ways I never thought possible. As the barriers to my past sexual trauma fell away, I found myself getting involved with new partners every few years.

With each new partner, I found myself facing the same fears and insecurities that stemmed from losing my father at the age of three. While I craved connection and intimacy, I also struggled to trust men. I constantly lived with the fear that if I truly opened myself up to love, I would once again be abandoned. My relationships brought both joy and pain as they forced me to confront my past trauma and push through my barriers to love.

There's a saying in the world of personal growth, "You teach what you need to know," and I became acutely aware that this was true for me. While I had become an expert in helping others navigate their sexual and intimacy issues, I realized I still had work to do on my own ability to form and maintain deep, lasting, romantic relationships.

## THE JOURNEY CONTINUES: CREATING INTIMACY RETREATS IN ASHEVILLE, NORTH CAROLINA

A combination of the wildfires in California and hating being so far away from my new grandson in Tennessee led me to my next adventure. After seven years of living and working in California, I felt a pull to return to the East Coast, closer to my roots and my growing family. But I didn't want to go back to the fast-paced life of New

York. Instead, I found myself drawn to the serene beauty of Asheville, North Carolina.

Asheville, with its misty mountains, vibrant arts scene, and community of healers and seekers, felt like it might be the perfect place for the next chapter of my life and work. When I spent the summer exploring Asheville, I felt a sense of peace and purpose wash over me. The lush green mountains and the crisp air of the Blue Ridge region seemed to breathe new life into my dreams and aspirations. I knew that this was where I was meant to create something truly special, but I wasn't exactly sure what that was.

After having dedicated a significant amount of time to working with individuals, I realized that my next focus would be on working with couples. I had worked with a small number of couples in California, and although I believed our work had been beneficial for them, I hadn't seen the level of change that I had hoped for. For me, weekly couples sessions felt like putting a Band-Aid on a gaping wound. The only exceptions to this were the few times when I did three-hour intensives. Those were powerful sessions that seemed very impactful.

That's when the idea for intimacy retreats began to take shape in my mind. What if I created an intensive, immersive way to help couples truly transform their relationships? I envisioned a safe, nurturing space where couples could step away from their daily lives and take a deep dive into healing and reconnecting—a place where they could learn new tools, explore their desires, and rediscover the spark that brought them together in the first place.

The concept excited me, but I also felt a twinge of anxiety. This was uncharted territory for me. Could I really create an experience that would transform relationships in just a few days? Doubt crept in, but I pushed it aside, reminding myself of how far I'd come and how many lives I'd already touched.

I found a beautiful property just outside the city, nestled in the Blue Ridge Mountains. It was perfect—secluded enough to provide privacy and a connection with nature, yet close enough to town for convenience. The split-level house was spacious, with enough space on the main floor for both my office and guest rooms, and the master suite extended out onto a large balcony complete with a hot tub!

Nestled on the lower level was a separate apartment, a hidden gem waiting to be discovered. I envisioned it as the perfect space for a rental retreat space catering to both couples attending an intimacy retreat and guests in search of an intimate, private sanctuary.

The suite would exude a sensual and alluring atmosphere, with dim lighting and plush, luxurious furnishings. Bold and seductive art pieces would adorn the walls, adding an element of passion to the space. At the center of the room would be a lavish king size canopy bed draped in twinkling lights for a touch of enchantment.

A sleek and newly renovated gourmet kitchen would sit off to the side, perfect for preparing tantalizing meals. And right outside the kitchen door, on the private deck, there would be a hot tub awaiting my guests with bubbling water and relaxing jets.

But perhaps the most intriguing feature would be the separate playroom, complete with low lighting and sensual materials scattered across a plush couch. And in one corner would hang a yoga swing, offering endless possibilities for pleasure and exploration. This was a space that would be designed for indulgence and sensuality, a haven for intimate moments and new experiences

The thought of creating this intimate space for others filled me with excitement and purpose. I could already imagine the satisfied smiles on my future guests' faces as they relaxed in this serene hideaway.

I spent months planning, researching, and developing the curriculum for these retreats. I wanted to create a perfect blend of education, experiential exercises, and relaxation. My goal was to give couples the tools they needed to communicate better, reignite their passion, and deepen their emotional and physical intimacy.

And so Passionate Intimacy Retreats was born, just as the pandemic struck! Thanks to some generous PPP loans from the government, my small start-up managed to stay afloat. And in truth, the timing couldn't have been better.

As the world slowly emerged from the grip of the pandemic, I found myself uniquely positioned to help couples navigate the new landscape of intimacy. Many had spent months in close quarters, their relationships tested by the stress and uncertainty of lockdowns. Some had grown closer, while others had drifted apart, realizing that the forced proximity had only highlighted existing issues. My phone began ringing off the hook with inquiries, and my calendar quickly filled up with carefully planned, socially-distanced private retreats.

One particularly memorable retreat was with Duncan and Stephanie, a couple in their early forties, who had only recently married and were struggling with intimacy and communication. They arrived at my doorstep, tension palpable between them. They told me they'd had a blowout fight the day before and had considered cancelling the retreat.

I immediately dropped my entire plan for our first afternoon, which is generally a gentle session to ease clients into the retreat and build trust and rapport with them. Instead we took a deep dive into their conflict, exploring the root causes of their communication breakdown.

As I listened to Duncan and Stephanie recount their argument, I could sense the pain and frustration beneath their words. It was clear that they both desperately wanted to connect, but years of misunderstandings and unmet needs had created a seemingly insurmountable wall between them.

"Let's try something different," I suggested, guiding them to sit facing each other on the comfortable outdoor couch. "I want you to look into each other's eyes, without speaking, for the next five minutes."

They both looked skeptical but agreed to try it. As they gazed at one another, I could see the subtle shifts in their expressions—flickers of tenderness, moments of vulnerability, and even flashes of the love that had brought them together in the first place.

When the timer went off, Stephanie had tears in her eyes. "I forgot how kind your eyes are," she whispered to Duncan. He reached out and took her hand.

That simple yet powerful exercise was the breakthrough we needed. Over the next three days, Duncan and Stephanie worked tirelessly to rebuild their connection. We explored communication and touch techniques, delved into their individual needs and desires, explored their sexual styles, and practiced vulnerability exercises that helped them rediscover the intimacy and physical connection they had lost.

On the final day of their retreat, as we sat on the deck overlooking the misty mountains, Stephanie turned to me with a smile. "I feel like we've fallen in love all over again," she said, her eyes glistening. Duncan nodded in agreement, pulling her close.

As I watched them leave, hand in hand, I felt a profound sense of fulfillment. This was why I had created this space, why I had embarked on this journey: I took it on to help people find their way back to each other, and to themselves.

Feeling settled in my home and my new business, I turned my attention to my own desire to find a new partner to share that delicious hot tub with. Three months after I moved to Asheville, I met Sam, a fellow Northern California transplant with a huge heart and spirit, who owned a "magic school bus" decked out with vibrant psychedelic art, a top-of-the-line sound system, and cozy beds for ultimate comfort and great sex.

We spent an amazing year together, taking turns quarantining in one of our houses, and he was by far the most skilled lover I'd ever had. That man knew how to use his hands and tongue and is the only person ever who has consistently been able to get me to orgasm through oral sex.

While Sam was committed to the long haul, I couldn't shake the feeling that this wasn't going to be the right relationship for me in the fullness of time. Deep down, I knew it wasn't meant to be forever. Also I was starting to get antsy and felt eager to venture out, socialize with new people, and discover all that Asheville had to offer as it slowly returned to normalcy.

I have a rule of thumb that when intense relationships end, I will remain essentially celibate for at least six months. It's an opportunity to allow my nervous system to settle back down, to process what I learned from the relationship, and to reconnect with myself before jumping into another one. So after Sam and I parted ways, I focused on nurturing myself and my business.

As the months passed, I found myself settling into a comfortable rhythm in Asheville. My retreat business was thriving, and I was making new friends in the vibrant community. But there was still a part of me that longed for a deep, lasting connection with a partner.

Although I was confident in my abilities as a sex and intimacy coach the world of online dating in 2021 was unfamiliar territory for me. So, towards the end of the year, I decided to hire a dating coach to help me navigate this new realm.

During our single session, she provided me with a helpful set of exercises to clarify my expectations and requirements for a partner. She also advised me on how to accurately portray myself in a dating profile. According to her, I should be open and transparent about my identity and desires in order to attract the right person. I took her advice and created a detailed dating profile on Spiritual Singles, which she had recommended.

Suffice it to say that did not go well. While I consider myself spiritual in many ways, the men on that site seemed to be looking for someone far more "woo-woo" than I am. I quickly realized I needed a different approach.

Luckily for me, my best friend in Asheville, who I'd met at a rally during my first visit there, is an energetic, spicy, forty-something with her finger on the pulse of the online dating scene. She helped me craft a fun and engaging profile, using each letter of the alphabet to describe myself:

*Asheville Newbie*

*Born to enjoy life*

*California transplant* and so on. (By the way, I highly recommend this approach to a dating profile...it got a huge number of responses).

We also uploaded some fun recent pictures, including a very sexy one of me dressed as a mermaid. I must confess, I lied about my age to appear younger and attract men in their fifties. I desired to date younger men who could keep up with my active lifestyle and high sexual energy.

At the start of 2022, I posted this profile on Bumble. The pickings were slim, especially in Asheville, with so many men holding up pictures of the fish they caught. It was enough to scare me away from online dating for the rest of my life. But just as I was getting ready to give up, I was matched with a very handsome, intelligent man who was a retired nurse.

His profile was witty and intriguing, with photos that showed a warm smile and kind eyes. We started messaging, and I was immediately drawn to his quick humor and thoughtful responses. After a few days of engaging conversation, we decided to meet for a walk in the park.

I arrived at our meeting place, my heart fluttering with a mix of excitement and nervousness. As he got out of his car to meet me, I was struck by how much more handsome he was in person. When he stood up to greet me, I noticed he was taller than I expected, with broad shoulders and a gentle demeanor.

"Hi, I'm Daren," he said, his voice warm and rich with a southern twang. "It's great to finally meet you in person."

Our walk turned into a three-hour conversation that flowed effortlessly. We talked about our past experiences, our hopes for the future, and our shared love of nature and adventure. Daren was fascinated by my work as a sex and intimacy coach, and it was clear from our conversation that he too was very sex positive and adventuresome.

As we strolled through the park, I felt a spark of connection with Daren that I hadn't experienced in a long time. His easy laugh and genuine interest in my work made me feel both seen and understood.

“I have to admit,” Daren said, a playful glint in his eye, “when I read your profile, I was intrigued. It's not every day you come across a sex and intimacy coach on a dating app.”

I chuckled, feeling a mix of pride and vulnerability. “Well, it's certainly an interesting conversation starter. But what about you? A retired nurse who's into Taoism and sex—that's quite the combination.”

Daren's face lit up. “Life's too short not to explore, right? I've always been fascinated by the connection between the body, mind, and spirit.”

At the end of our date I confessed to Daren that I was actually ten years his senior. I braced myself for his reaction, expecting disappointment or perhaps even anger at my deception. But to my surprise, he simply smiled and said, "Well, you certainly don't look or act your age. And honestly, I'm even more impressed now."

His response filled me with relief and a renewed sense of excitement. We agreed to meet again soon, and as I watched him drive away, I felt a flutter of hope in my chest. Could this be the start of something special?

For a week, I took refuge from the harsh winter in Florida, while staying in constant contact with Daren through talking and texting. Our free evenings were occupied by watching his favorite series, Sex and the City, via Zoom. It was refreshing to be with someone who knew the show inside out and could give me detailed explanations of each episode before they even aired.

On a total whim, I invited him to come to Florida for the weekend, and much to my delight and surprise, he agreed without hesitation. As I waited for him at the airport, I felt a mix of excitement and nervousness. Would our connection be as strong in person as it was over the phone and video calls?

When Daren walked through the arrivals gate, all my doubts melted away. His face lit up with a warm smile as he spotted me, and he enveloped me in a tight hug. The chemistry between us was palpable, and we could barely keep our hands off each other as we made our way to my rented condo.

That weekend was a whirlwind of passion, laughter, and deep conversation. We explored the beaches, tried local restaurants, and spent hours talking about our lives, dreams, and desires. Daren's openness and curiosity about my work as a sex and intimacy coach led to some incredibly intimate and vulnerable moments between us.

Our flight home together is etched in my memory forever; we held hands for the entire journey. Tears of joy streamed down my face as I felt I had finally found the person I had been searching for all my life.

My intuition proved to be correct; I had experienced the phenomenon of love at first sight. It was not without its rough patches, but four years later, we are happily living together, intertwined in each other's existence. Our days are filled with inside jokes and shared experiences, our nights spent wrapped in each other's embrace.

Our relationship isn't just passionate; it is deeply nurturing, supportive, and growth-oriented. We challenge each other, learn from each other, and continually find new ways to deepen our connection.

Daren is not only an incredible partner, he is also my cheerleader and confidante. He is the one with whom I share my fears about a particular couple I'm working with, my frustrations if I feel like I'm not on my game during a retreat, and my celebrations and successes when couples leave my retreat so much healthier and more connected than when they arrived. He also has been urging me for some time to write another book. I am deeply grateful for his loving "kick in the ass," because he realized that if I could just start writing, the pages would flow. And of course, he was right about that.

The first thing I did was to call up my amazing publisher Brenda Knight, who is now at the helm of her own publishing company, *Books That Save Lives.* When I pitched my idea for a book for couples about sex and intimacy, Brenda was fully on board without any hesitations. And so *The Sex and Intimacy Repair Kit* was born.

# 2

# HOW DID WE GET HERE? WHY COUPLES STRUGGLE AND END UP IN SEXLESS RELATIONSHIPS

Jess and Henry were sitting in my office on opposite ends of the couch. They were recounting for me how they had met in their first year of college. I asked Henry what attracted him to Jess. “It was her laugh,” he said, “she had this big, genuine, musical laugh, and she always was able to find the lightness in any situation. But I haven’t heard her laugh like that in years.”

Jess looked down and played with the fringe on her sweater. “We were so in love in the beginning. I felt like Henry was my best friend and an amazing lover. I could share anything with him, and our future looked so promising”.

“What do you think happened over the past thirty years?” I asked gently; “How did you get to this place?” Jess paused, her fingers still twirling the fringe. “Life happened, I suppose,” she said softly. "We got caught up in our careers, raising the kids, paying the mortgage, taking care of our aging parents. Somewhere along the way, we became roommates and co-managers of our household.”

Henry nodded, a pained expression crossing his face. “I remember the day I realized I couldn't remember the last time we'd had a real conversation—not about schedules or bills, but about our dreams and fears. It scared me.”

“And yet you're both here now. What made you decide to come to an intimacy retreat?”

Jess looked up, her eyes meeting Henry's for the first time since they'd entered my office. “Our youngest left for college last month,” she said. “Suddenly, the house was so quiet. And in that quiet, I realized I barely knew the man I was living with.”

Henry added, “We’re in our early fifties and healthy, and this is not the relationship either of us wants. Things either need to drastically improve or we both need to move on.”

I nodded, sensing the mix of determination and apprehension in Henry's voice. “That's a brave realization,” I said. “Many couples struggle to admit when they've reached that crossroads.”

Jess shifted on the couch, turning slightly towards Henry. “I think...I think we both want to try,” she said, her voice barely above a whisper. “But I'm scared. What if we can't find our way back to each other?”

Henry reached across the couch, his hand hovering uncertainly in the space between them. After a moment's hesitation, Jess reached out and took it.

“I'm scared too,” Henry admitted. “But I remember that girl with the infectious laugh. And I remember the guy who could make her laugh. I want to believe they're still in there somewhere.”

I watched as they held hands, a small but significant move towards connection.

This pattern is all too common when working with couples struggling with intimacy. It begins like any fairytale: Two people meet, fall in love, and start building a life together. But as time passes, external pressures and responsibilities take over, leaving little time for nurturing their relationship. As a result, physical intimacy fades into the background, becoming less and less frequent until it disappears completely. And before they know it, they find themselves trapped in a relationship without passion or emotional connection. This heartbreaking story is unfortunately all too common.

Statistically, 7 percent of couples have not had sex in the past year and 15 percent have had very little sex (i.e., two to three times per year).

But if one defines a sexless marriage as having sex less than ten times per year, that percentage jumps up to 20 percent. However, most couples counselors would dispute that number, given how prevalent sexless marriages are in our practices. Gen Z is even having less sex than previous generations, with over 25 percent in a recent study reporting that they have never experienced partnered sex.

Given all this data, it's fair to say that we are experiencing an epidemic of sexless relationships in this country.

In this chapter, we will explore the common challenges that often plague couples like Jess and Henry and leave them emotionally and sexually unsatisfied. These struggles can lead to a lack of intimacy and fulfillment in the bedroom. We will identify these obstacles and provide solutions for overcoming them in later chapters, ultimately creating a stronger and more satisfying bond between you and your partner.

## Inadequate or Poor Communication

It is a universal truth that the vast majority of relationship problems stem from issues with communication. These problems can range from expecting your partner to anticipate your thoughts and needs to fearing judgment if you express your true emotions. The intricacies of effective communication are like a maze filled with hidden obstacles and potential misinterpretations. It takes skill and effort to successfully navigate this maze, but doing so is essential for a healthy and fulfilling relationship. Failure to communicate openly and honestly can lead to misunderstandings and resentment, ultimately damaging the bond between two people.

In my years of counseling couples, I've found that communication breakdowns often stem from fear—fear of vulnerability, fear of rejection, fear of judgment, or fear of conflict.

**Case Study: Jane and Whitt**

Jane and Whitt had been married for over twenty years—a second marriage for both of them—and they were struggling with intimacy and emotional connection. "The biggest issue in my mind," said Jane, "is that ever since Whitt's company was taken over by a national conglomerate, he's been working sixty to seventy hours a week. By the time he rolls in at seven or eight at night, he's exhausted and just wants to sleep."

Whitt nodded, his shoulders slumping. "I know it's been tough on Jane," he said. "But I feel like I don't have a choice. The new management is demanding, and I'm constantly worried about job security. If I can just do this for a few more years, we'll be able to retire more comfortably."

Jane sighed, her frustration evident. "I understand that, Whitt. But it feels like you're proving your worth to them at the expense of our relationship. Besides, I'm making more money now since my promotion, and I just don't understand why you can't pull back your hours! This is the first time in three years that you've taken any time off."

I leaned forward, addressing them both. "It sounds like you both have really strong feelings about your circumstances but haven't been able to talk about them with each other. Jane, you're feeling very lonely and miss being able to spend quality time with Whitt."

Tears started streaming down Jane's face. "I'm so scared that he's going to have a heart attack...he's under so much pressure...I'm so afraid of losing him."

"Whitt, how does it make you feel to hear Jane express those fears?" I gently asked.

Whitt's eyes widened, a look of surprise crossing his face. He turned to Jane, his voice soft. "I had no idea you were so worried about my health. I...I guess I've been so focused on providing for our future, I didn't realize how much I was neglecting our present."

Jane wiped her eyes, her voice trembling. "I don't want a comfortable retirement if it means losing you now, Whitt. I want us to enjoy our life together now, while we're still young and healthy enough to do so."

Whitt reached out, taking Jane's hand. "I'm sorry, Jane. I've been so caught up in my own stress and fears about work, I didn't see how it was affecting you. I don't want to lose us either."

"Whitt," I gently prodded, "I hear you're concerned about not being able to provide for your retirement, but I'm wondering if maybe there's something more going on here for you? When you think about no longer working, what shows up for you?"

Whitt paused, his brow furrowing as he considered my question. "I...I guess I've never really thought about it that way," he said slowly. "Work has always been such a big part of who I am. The idea of not working, of not having that purpose..." He trailed off, looking suddenly vulnerable.

Jane gently squeezed his hand, encouraging him to continue.

“I suppose," Whitt said, his voice barely above a whisper, "I'm afraid of losing my identity—of not being needed anymore. My whole life, I've defined myself by my career, by being the provider. Without that, who am I?”

I nodded, understanding dawning. “So, it's not just about financial security, is it? It's about maintaining your sense of identity and worth.”

“Yes,” Whitt said, looking relieved. Jane looked at him, surprise evident on her face. “But Whitt, there are so many other opportunities for you to explore after you retire. You can volunteer, you can even start your own consulting business, and my job is flexible, so we can do more traveling.”

Whitt's eyes lit up at Jane's words. “You're right,” he said, a hint of excitement creeping into his voice. “I've always wanted to mentor young entrepreneurs. And remember that woodworking class we took together years ago? I've been thinking about getting back into that.”

Jane smiled, her first genuine smile since they'd entered my office. “I remember. You were so good at it. You made that beautiful jewelry box for my birthday.”

I watched as a moment of connection passed between them, a small spark reigniting. “It sounds like you both have lots of feelings and thoughts about the future that you haven't shared with each other in a while,” I observed. “What would it be like to start having those conversations and to really listen to each other?”

Jane and Whitt exchanged glances, mixed hope and uncertainty in their eyes.

“I think...I think that would be good,” Jane said softly. “I miss those conversations we used to have, dreaming about our future together.”

Whitt nodded, squeezing Jane's hand. "Me too. I've been so caught up in my own head, I forgot how much I enjoyed just talking with you, sharing our hopes and fears."

"That's an excellent starting point," I affirmed. "Communication is key to rebuilding intimacy. But it's not just about talking more—it's about learning to truly listen and understand each other."

I leaned forward, addressing them both. "For your first exercise, I want you to set aside time every evening—even if it's just fifteen minutes—to talk without distractions: no phones, no TV, just the two of you. Make sure these check-ins are not about the routine of your lives, but rather share feelings, fears, and hopes."

When Whitt and Jane came back the next day, they were smiling and holding hands. "Wow," I exclaimed, "you seem like a totally different couple from yesterday."

Jane beamed, her eyes sparkling with newfound energy. "It's amazing what a difference a day can make," she said. "Last night, we had our first check-in like you suggested. We sat out on the porch after dinner, and it felt like we were dating again."

Whitt nodded enthusiastically. "We talked for hours, way past our usual bedtime. I can't remember the last time we did that."

"What was that experience like for each of you?" I asked, curious to hear more.

Jane's expression softened. "It was...liberating. I realized how much I'd been holding back, afraid to burden Whitt with my worries. But once I started talking, it all came pouring out."

Whitt reached over and squeezed Jane's hand. "And I listened, really listened, for the first time in a long time. We even began to brainstorm a plan for me to cut back on my hours and slowly transition towards retirement."

"Fantastic, I said. "I love that you were able to communicate openly with each other. You're a great team, and I'm confident you can work through this together."

## Unresolved Conflicts and Resentments

Many relationship struggles stem from unresolved conflicts and resentments that have built up over long periods of time. Whether it's with a romantic partner, business colleague, family member, or friend, conflicts are bound to occur at times. How you handle these conflicts can either foster a healthy relationship or allow toxicity to seep in and over time create intimacy issues.

Unresolved conflicts, misunderstandings, and miscommunications can lead to a buildup of resentment within a relationship. Sometimes, these conflicts are not even recognized by your partner. For example, your partner may respond to your question in a condescending tone that hurts your feelings. Instead of addressing it and risking an argument, you choose to ignore it and move on. However, these little incidents can accumulate over time and result in a larger issue as resentment continues to build up.

Resentment can also fester and grow in a relationship when conflicts arise and both partners are aware of it. These issues can range from how seemingly insignificant tasks are handled, like forgetting to take out the trash on time, to more significant events, such as forgetting your partner's birthday or anniversary. The tension builds up like a volcano, with each small issue adding to the simmering resentment between you and your partner until it's like a ticking time bomb, waiting to explode at any moment.

In most cases, conflicts among couples are not properly addressed and resolved. Many do not possess the necessary tools to effectively repair conflicts, and instead often resort to simply ignoring them.

Even in cases where a couple tries to repair a conflict, they often do so too quickly and incompletely, leading to feelings of frustration and invalidation for one or both partners.

Resentment can also arise when one partner feels they are carrying the bulk of the emotional, physical, or mental load in the relationship without their efforts being acknowledged. For example, if you consistently feel like your needs for affection, quality time, or sex are being neglected, you might start to harbor resentment. Over time, even small slights or disappointments can compound, leading to a deep sense of frustration and bitterness.

Resentment thrives in silence. When you don't express these feelings in a healthy way, you internalize the hurt. This leads to emotional shutdown, passive-aggressive behavior, or even outright hostility, further damaging the relationship. The emotional disconnection often results in reduced sexual desire because you feel too hurt, angry, or distant to engage in intimacy.

## LACK OF EMOTIONAL CONNECTION AND FEAR OF BEING VULNERABLE

One of my favorite T-shirts has this written on the front of it: "Vulnerability is sexy." Yet most people are terrified of being vulnerable. But vulnerability is the glue that creates and holds an emotional connection together and allows intimacy to flourish.

**Case Study: Sarah and Mike**

Meet Sarah and Mike, who have been married for fifteen years. On the surface, they had it all—successful careers in New York City, two beautiful children, and a spacious home in the suburbs.

Sarah's words echoed in my mind: "We're like two ships passing in the night. We coexist, we parent together, but we don't really connect anymore."

Mike nodded, his expression a mix of frustration and sadness. "I feel like I don't even know how to talk to Sarah anymore. Every conversation feels like it could turn into an argument."

I moved in closer, addressing them both. "It sounds like you've both been feeling disconnected for a while. Can you tell me more about when you first noticed this distance growing between you?"

Sarah sighed, her fingers twisting the ring on her left hand. "I think it started gradually, after our second child was born. We were both so busy with work and the kids, we just...stopped making time for each other."

Mike nodded, his brow furrowed. "I remember feeling like we were just going through the motions: wake up, get the kids ready, go to work, come home, eat dinner, put the kids to bed, repeat. There was no...us time anymore."

"And how did that make you feel?" I prompted gently.

Sarah's eyes welled up with tears. "Lonely. So incredibly lonely. Even when we were in the same room, it felt like Mike was a hundred miles away."

"You never made any time for me Sarah," Mike interjected. "Every time I tried to initiate sex, you turned me down. You were always too tired or too busy, or you had something else more important to do. So I just stopped trying."

Sarah's eyes flashed with hurt and anger. "That's not fair, Mike. You know how exhausted I was, working full-time and taking care of two young children. I needed your help and support, not just physical intimacy."

Mike's jaw clenched. "I was working long hours too, Sarah. I felt like nothing I did was ever good enough for you."

I held up a hand, gently interrupting their rising voices. “I hear a lot of pain and frustration from both of you. It sounds like you've both been feeling unseen and unappreciated for a long time.”

They both fell silent, the tension in the room palpable.

“Sarah, Mike,” I said softly, “what I'm hearing is that you both desperately want to connect with each other, but you're afraid of being hurt or rejected. It also sounds like you’re both unable to talk vulnerably with each other about your feelings.”

“Talking about my emotions isn’t something I’m very good at,” said Mike. “Half the time I’m not even sure what I’m feeling.”

“That's very common,” I said, offering a reassuring smile. “Many people struggle with identifying and expressing their emotions, especially if they weren't encouraged to do so growing up. But it's a skill that can be learned and practiced.”

Sarah looked at Mike, her expression softening slightly. “I didn't realize you felt that way. I guess I've been so focused on my own frustrations, I didn't see how much you were struggling too.”

Mike met her gaze, vulnerability flickering in his eyes. “I...I'm sorry, Sarah. I know I haven't been the most emotionally available husband. I want to be better at this, for you and for us.”

I smiled, sensing a small breakthrough. “That's a great start, both of you. Recognizing and acknowledging each other's struggles is the first step towards rebuilding your emotional connection.”

## The Stress of Life

There is no doubt that stress is one of the leading reasons that couples struggle with their sex life. It seeps into every aspect of their being, both emotionally and physically. Like a powerful storm, stress unleashes a torrent of cortisol, flooding the body and leaving one feeling jittery and tense. In this state, even the thought of intimacy can feel overwhelming and unattainable. The effects of stress on the mind and body can create a perfect storm of disaster when it comes to sexual desire and satisfaction.

Unfortunately, life seems to have become even more stressful in the last decade. The demands of work, with its unrelenting 24/7 barrage of emails and texts, the high cost of living and economic pressures while striving just to make ends meet, and the fearmongering and pressure we feel from the news and social media have created a level of stress and intensity in our lives that is unsustainable. In addition, many couples are also perfectly situated in the sandwich generation, dealing with both raising children and taking care of aging parents. As a society, we are burning the candle at both ends, and there is very little left for ourselves and our relationships.

Along with stress, a lack of adequate sleep will also negatively impact intimacy. The silence of a bedroom devoid of intimacy, filled only with the sounds of tossing and turning from restless sleep, can create a feeling of distance and disconnection between partners. Lack of good sleep can also leave you irritable and short-tempered, increasing the odds of an argument or conflict arising—a definite intimacy killer.

## Mismatched Sexual Desires

If you were to survey a group of sex therapists, they would tell you that a mismatch in sexual desires is the most common problem that their clients face. What this typically looks like is that one partner (often the female in a hetero couple) is less interested in sex than the other. I also see this happen with lesbian couples, so it is not necessarily a sexual preference issue.

While I don't disagree with my sex therapist colleagues per se, I do believe there's a chicken and egg problem here. Does the mismatched desire cause the physical intimacy issues, or is it the lack of emotional intimacy that creates the mismatched desire?

As you will learn in Part 3 of this book, the pathways for sexual arousal for women and men can be vastly different. Since it is women who are most often the low desire partner in a couple, it is worth spending some time on understanding the intricacies of women's desire. For an in-depth analysis of women's challenges around their sexual desire, I highly recommend you read my book, *Living an Orgasmic Life*, or sign up for my online class, "Reclaiming Your Desire."

Women's desire and libido are multifaceted and complex. If it was simple to diagnose and treat, we would already have a Viagra equivalent for women. Instead, we have short-term treatments, such as the "O shot" and a generally recognized ineffective drug called "Addy" which has significant side effects and must be taken daily.

The truth is that there are myriad reasons why women struggle with their sexual desire. They include body dysmorphia, sexual shame, hormonal fluctuations, trauma and sexual abuse, feeling emotionally disconnected from their partner, going through pain during sex, never experiencing pleasure and orgasms, and not having their core desires met. Neuroscientist Louann Brezendine, author of *The Female Brain*, has shown how fluctuations in hormones across a woman's lifespan can also profoundly influence desire. Recognizing these shifts can help couples meet each other with compassion and flexibility.

However, when talking about mismatched desires, it's important to understand that there are two different kinds of desire: spontaneous desire and responsive desire. While both women and men experience both, spontaneous desire is more common in men, while responsive desire is more typical for women, especially as we age.

Spontaneous desire is what most people think of as "normal" desire —it's when you suddenly feel aroused and want sex, seemingly out of nowhere. Responsive desire, on the other hand, only kicks in after arousal activity has started. A person with responsive desire may not feel "in the mood" initially but can become aroused once things get going.

This difference can create challenges in relationships. The partner with spontaneous desire may feel rejected when their advances are not reciprocated. Meanwhile, the partner with responsive desire may feel pressured or inadequate for not initiating or wanting sex as often. But as Emily Nagoski so beautifully explains in her book *Come as You Are*, understanding the differences between spontaneous and responsive desire helps couples to stop blaming themselves and instead recognize these are normal variations in arousal.

**Case Study: Melissa and James**

Take Melissa and James, for example. They came to me struggling with mismatched desires that were creating tension in their ten-year marriage.

"I just don't understand," James said, frustration evident in his voice. "We used to have such an active sex life, we would have sex four to five times a week. Now I'm lucky if we have sex twice a month." Melissa looked down, her cheeks flushing. "It's not that I don't love James or find him attractive," she said softly. "I just...I never seem to feel in the mood anymore. By the time we get to bed, I'm exhausted from work and taking care of the kids. Sex is the last thing on my mind."

James sighed, running a hand through his hair. "I try to initiate, but Melissa always has an excuse. It makes me feel unwanted, like she's not attracted to me anymore."

I nodded, understanding their frustration. "What you're describing is actually quite common," I explained. "Melissa, it sounds like you may have more of a responsive desire pattern, while James has more spontaneous desire. I'm guessing that when you do actually start having sex, you start enjoying it. Correct?" Melissa nodded, "Yes, once James starts touching and kissing me, I start to relax and feel turned on. I just struggle with getting started."

James looked surprised. "I had no idea," he said softly. "I thought you just weren't interested anymore."

I smiled encouragingly at them both. "This is a great breakthrough. Understanding each other's desire patterns is crucial. James, knowing that Melissa's desire is responsive can help you approach intimacy differently."

"Tell me more," said James, looking at her with interest.

"Well," I explained, "instead of waiting for Melissa to initiate or expecting her to be immediately ready for sex, you could focus on creating an atmosphere that allows her desire to build. This might mean starting with nonsexual touch, like a light massage, and creating an environment that allows her to relax. Low lights, sexy music, maybe even inviting her into a bath."

"I would love that," said Melissa, gently squeezing James' arm. "The few instances when we've taken our time have been so much more enjoyable for me."

"But Melissa," I gently prodded, "initiating sex can't always be James' responsibility. That will also eventually create tension in the relationship."

James nodded, "I'm so afraid of being rejected that sometimes I won't even try."

"To cope with this in my own relationship, I constantly remind myself that Daren's touch will inevitably lead to my body responding. That's why I make a conscious effort to initiate some form of sensual contact at least once a week, even if I'm not particularly in the mood for it."

Melissa nodded slowly, taking in my words. "I can see how that would help," she said. "I guess I've been so caught up in feeling guilty about not being 'in the mood' that I didn't even consider initiating when I wasn't feeling desire."

I moved forward, addressing them both. "It's important to remember that desire naturally fluctuates over the course of a relationship. What worked for you in the beginning might not work now, and that's okay. The key is to keep communicating and adapting together." They looked at each other with understanding, compassion, and a new sense of hope.

Now that we've explored the common blocks that trip couples up around intimacy—resentment, stress, time pressures, and poor communication—it's clear that most relationship disconnection isn't about lack of love, but lack of emotional safety and understanding. In the next chapter, we'll begin to unpack what true intimacy actually looks and feels like. Creating connection isn't just about spending more time together—it's about presence, attunement, and the willingness to be vulnerable. Real intimacy begins when we slow down enough to truly see and be seen.

# 3

# IN-TO-ME-SEE: UNDERSTANDING THE ROOTS OF CONNECTION

The word "intimacy" can mean different things to different people. When men talk about it, they often use it as a euphemism for sex. On the other hand, when women discuss intimacy, they usually mean emotional closeness and connection. This difference in interpretation can lead to misunderstandings between partners. Both are seeking intimacy, but from two completely different, yet related, perspectives.

**Case Study: Connie and Jay**

Like most of the couples who reach out to me, Connie and Jay were struggling in their marriage. They clearly loved each other, but they both felt that something was missing.

Jay craved more physical connection and touch. He lamented that their sex life over the last five years had been reduced to "once a month, if I'm lucky and all the stars are aligned for Connie." Connie was similarly frustrated. She felt emotionally disconnected from Jay. She longed for deeper conversations and felt closed off from Jay when he didn't communicate his feelings. "I just want to feel close to him again," she told me, her eyes welling with tears. "But every time we start to connect, he immediately tries to turn it into sex."

As I began to delve deeper into their relationship, it became clear that while both Connie and Jay wanted more intimacy, their definitions and expectations were misaligned. Jay, like many men, experiences emotional closeness through physical intimacy; thus sex becomes the doorway to a deeper emotional bond with his partner. For Connie, like many women, feeling emotionally connected to their partner is the aphrodisiac that fuels their desire for sex.

During one particularly revealing moment, Jay admitted, "I initiate sex because I want to feel close to Connie. When she turns me down, I feel rejected and unloved." Connie's eyes widened with surprise. "I had no idea," she said softly, gently reaching out for Jay's hand.

This moment illustrates one of the most common themes that I encounter when helping couples navigate relationship challenges: failure to effectively communicate about their needs and desires. This lack of communication inevitably leads to a sense of detachment between partners, creating a growing chasm in their connection.

Without open and honest communication, the relationship bond becomes strained and begins to fray, leaving them both feeling alone and misunderstood. It is a familiar pattern, repeating itself over and over, until eventually fissures show up in the foundation of the relationship.

Once I pointed out the misunderstanding to Connie and Jay, I asked Connie to turn towards Jay and clarify what intimacy means to her. "Intimacy is when I feel connected to you. You open up and share your emotions with me without hesitation. I enjoy snuggling with you and discussing our day. Most importantly, I want to know that you truly see me."

I asked Jay and Connie to continue to look at each other and allow me to speak on behalf of each of them to help them access their deeper unsaid emotions. This is a unique and powerful tool that I've learned from "Attachment University," created by my friend and mentor Derek Hart.

"When we're disconnected, I feel so lonely and sad. I really miss you, Jay. When I don't know how to reach you, I'm afraid that I'm losing you. Sometimes I feel so alone in our relationship."

"I had no idea you felt that way," I spoke on behalf of Jay. "For me, intimacy is about feeling desired and wanted. When we're physically close, I feel loved and connected to you. But when you turn away or seem uninterested, I feel rejected and alone too."

As Connie looked into Jay's eyes, tears began to flow, and Jay reached out to comfort Connie. I felt Jay softening as they shared a moment of true vulnerability and understanding. This was the beginning of true intimacy.

## IN-TO-ME-SEE

The need for intimacy and connection is a fundamental human desire, as seen in Maslow's Hierarchy of Needs, a psychological theory that posits human motivation progresses through five levels —from basic physiological survival needs, like food and safety, to higher-level needs for love, esteem, and ultimately, self-actualization. Sex is at the bottom of the pyramid, along with food, shelter, and water and it also shows up on the third level of love and belonging. Human beings are wired for connection. We crave understanding, acceptance, and love from others. This deep-seated need for intimacy is at the core of our most meaningful relationships.

The phrase "in-to-me-see" beautifully captures the essence of true intimacy. It's an invitation to allow another person to see into your innermost self—your hopes, fears, dreams, and vulnerabilities. It's about being fully present and transparent with your partner, creating a safe space where both of you can be your authentic selves without fear of judgment or rejection.

For Connie and Jay, their journey towards true intimacy was just beginning. As they continued their sessions with me, they learned to peel back the layers of miscommunication and misunderstanding that had built up over the years. They practiced active listening, transparency, and empathy—key components of emotional intimacy.

## Active Listening

Active listening is the cornerstone of good communication. It is the practice of fully concentrating on, understanding, responding to, and remembering what your partner is saying. It's more than just hearing words—it involves engaging with your partner emotionally and intellectually, ensuring they feel seen and heard.

Key components of active listening include:

- Being Present: Give your partner your undivided attention.
- Nonverbal Cues: Use body language such as nodding and maintaining eye contact.
- Reflective Responses: Paraphrase or summarize what your partner has said to confirm understanding.
- Empathy: Validate your partner's feelings without trying to fix or judge their experience.
- Avoid Interruptions: Allow your partner to express their thoughts fully before responding.

## *Active Listening Exercise*

Though this method will be most useful in resolving conflicts and relationship repair conversations, I highly recommend starting with non-relationship matters such as a work incident or issues with family or friends. It's easier to practice active listening when there's no chance of setting off each other's triggers, since feeling triggered can make it almost impossible to fully listen when your nervous system is on high alert.

1. Set the Stage:
Find a quiet space and set aside 10–15 minutes.
2. Choose Roles:
One partner is the speaker, the other is the listener.

*Speaker's Role:*
Share thoughts or feelings using "I" statements (example: "I feel overwhelmed at work").
Keep it concise and focused.

*Listener's Role:*
Listen without interrupting, judging, or trying to fix anything.
Reflect back what you heard with empathy (example: "It sounds like work has been very demanding lately. That must be really challenging for you right now.")
Be very present and stay in eye contact with the speaker.

*Switch Roles:*
Check in with the speaker to assess whether they felt understood. If they didn't, then the Listener should ask the speaker what would help them feel more understood (consider if it would help to rephrase, or if the body language not aligned with the words).
After the speaker feels understood, trade roles and repeat.

3. Wrap-Up:
Discuss how it felt to be heard and what you learned about each other. If something didn't work (for example, you felt your partner didn't really reflect back what you said, tried to fix something, or imposed their own meaning), share that information. These are all common pitfalls when you start to practice active listening.

## Transparency

In the intimate space of a romantic relationship, true transparency requires absolute honesty with your partner about every aspect of your life. It means laying bare your financial situation, both past and present, and being open about any lingering wounds or scars from previous relationships. It also involves expressing your needs and desires without fear or hesitation.

Transparency is not easy for most couples as it can unearth feelings of shame, unworthiness, fear of vulnerability, and even jealousy when discussing financial matters or past romantic entanglements. But in order to build a strong and trusting bond, complete openness is essential. It's like stripping away layers of fabric to reveal the raw and vulnerable core beneath.

## Empathy

Empathy is the ability to deeply understand and share the feelings, experiences, and perspectives of another person. It asks you to put aside all of your own judgments and stories and literally stand in your partner's shoes. Some people are naturally very empathetic, while for others, cultivating empathy can be very awkward and challenging.

But empathy is one of the most critical components to building emotional connection and closeness. It allows you to truly see and hear each other without judgment, fostering a safe space for vulnerability and honesty. Empathy helps bridge misunderstandings, validate emotions, and create a sense of being deeply valued and supported.

As Connie and Jay continued their work with me, they began to practice these skills of active listening, transparency, and empathy in their daily lives. It wasn't always easy—old habits die hard, and there were moments of frustration and backsliding. But slowly and steadily, they began to build a new foundation for their relationship. Connie recounted this conversation with Jay a few months into our session.

One evening, Connie came home from work visibly upset. In the past, Jay might have tried to immediately fix the problem or brush it off, which would have completely invalidated Connie's feelings and caused her to build up more resentment. This time, however, he took a deep breath and remembered our discussions on active listening.

"Connie, you seem upset. Do you want to talk about it?" he asked, giving her his full attention.

Connie hesitated for a moment, then nodded. She began to share about a difficult colleague at work who continued to undermine her, expressing her fears about job security and her feelings of inadequacy. Jay listened intently, maintained eye contact, and nodded in agreement.

When she was finished speaking, Jay reflected on what he heard. "Ouch, Connie, that sounds really hard. That must be so frustrating for you that it keeps on happening. I know how much you care about your work. I'm so sorry."

Connie's eyes welled up with tears. "Yes, thank you for really listening and understanding."

As she related this story, Connie told me that this was the first time in their marriage that she truly felt seen and heard by Jay.

Jay's gaze shifted between the two of us, and he confessed, "I struggled to resist solving this problem for Connie, but it was worth it to see her soften during our conversation. It brought us closer." Connie looked at Jay and gave him a sweet kiss. As the weeks went by, these moments of connection became more frequent.

## *Empathetic Listening Exercise:*

This practice builds upon the active listening exercise. It is also one of the key components of the relationship repair process that you will learn later in this book.

Again, I strongly urge you to choose non-relationship issues when starting out, just as Connie and Jay did as they practiced in our case study above.

Follow the steps for the Active Listening Exercise from a few pages back. When you come to the part of the Listener's role of reflecting back with empathy, add the following elements.

1. The Listener reflects back with empathy.
2. The Speaker listens carefully and considers whether the empathy landed or whether they even felt empathy from their partner.
3. The Listener suggests to their partner what they would really like to hear that would make them feel seen and understood.
4. The Speaker tries again until the Listener feels that empathy has been authentically expressed.
5. Switch Roles
6. Debrief and Discuss

While this exercise seems simple, it is actually one of the most challenging exercises that I teach couples. Because so many people have a hard time expressing empathy, do not be surprised if the Speaker does not feel any empathy coming from the Listener the first time around.

Sometimes the Listener will say all the right words, but the empathy still doesn't land because of their tone of voice. It's perfectly fine to ask your partner to soften their voice or to maintain eye contact. Less is more when it comes to expressing empathy. Words that I often suggest include simple phrases like "That sounds really hard," "That must have really felt awful," or "I can see how hurt you are."

Body language is also very important when authentically expressing empathy. A touch on the arm, nodding, and showing through your eyes that you feel their pain will often go a long way towards giving your partner the sense that you truly understand and empathize with their feelings.

## THE THREE STAGES OF SEXUAL RELATIONSHIPS

In order to understand how to create passionate intimacy, we first need to examine the different stages of sexual relationships. As you read this section, begin to consider where you would put your relationship on the spectrum described below. It's also important to understand that not all couples go through all these stages and that many sexual challenges arise because the relationship is stuck in the first or second stage.

### Stage 1: New Relationship Energy & Friction Sex

We've all experienced the intensity and excitement of "new relationship energy," also known as the *limerence* stage. Many couples who attend my retreats express their desire to rekindle the passion and desire they had in the early stages of their relationship.

Think back on the early days of your relationship. If you're anything like me, you were in the throes of passion and couldn't seem to get enough of each other. The sight of your partner entering the room not only sparked excitement in your eyes, but also in your genitals. Sex was often wild and unbridled, happening frequently without hesitation or boundaries, allowing for experimentation and discovery.

New relationship energy is actually fueled by hormones creating the sense of attraction and desire. In her book, *Why We Love: The Nature and Chemistry of Romantic Love*, researcher Helen Fisher examined what happens to our brains in the early stages of love. The euphoria, excitement, and rush that you feel are related to shifts in our brain chemistry. Dopamine (the addiction hormone) increases, as does norepinephrine (the high energy rush hormone).

These hormones light up the amygdala—the pleasure center in the brain—causing you to crave more connection, more contact with your partner, and more sex. It's Mother Nature's way of moving us toward procreating the species. These hormones are so plentiful and strong that they can sometimes override trauma, which is why it's not uncommon for some individuals who have experienced sexual trauma to find themselves seemingly trauma-free in the beginning of a new relationship. Unfortunately, when the limerence period ends, typically within six to eighteen months, the trauma usually resurfaces, causing confusion and distress for both partners.

During this initial stage, sex is often driven by friction and physical sensation. The focus is primarily on genital stimulation and achieving orgasm. While this can be exciting and pleasurable, it tends to be more surface level and lacking in the deeper emotional connection that develops in later stages.

This stage is generally unsustainable because it has diminishing returns. It can become rote and boring, and especially for women, can cause them to lose desire since it lacks emotional safety. It can be maintained for long periods of time with the use of drugs and alcohol. The need for a glass of wine or two before sex is indicative of a couple being stuck in this stage. It also lays the groundwork for sex to become performative, genitally focused, and orgasm and goal oriented.

## STAGE 2: VALIDATION SEX

Once the new relationship energy ends, you move into the phase of sex being used to test the strength of the relationship and your partner's loyalty and level of commitment. This stage is fraught with challenges and causes many couples to shift into patterns of obligatory or sexless relationships.

In this stage, you begin to form an attachment to your partner. However, the attachment also comes with the fear and anxiety of losing them. You are constantly asking yourself whether your partner cares for and loves you and looking for signs and indicators, and you use physical intimacy as a way to seek reassurance and confirm your partner's commitment.

This fear of loss prevents both partners from taking risks. Women may hold back from asking for what they want or providing feedback, fearing that displeasing their partner may chase them away. Men may fear expressing their genuine sexual desires and fantasies, which could lead to the possibility of being rejected and scaring their partner away. The lack of vulnerability and emotional connection can perpetuate this cycle for years.

Couples stuck in the validation sex phase may end up in a sexless relationship or with sex having become a chore, something to check off the to-do list. The emotional disconnection and lack of vulnerability often lead to resentment, with one or both partners feeling unfulfilled and undesired. Very often all the emotional anxiety associated with one partner pursuing sex and the other retreating results in a couple choosing just to hold hands and cuddle, which continues to validate the relationship without the anxiety involved in sex. Another frequent outcome is for sex to become routine and boring, leading to one or both partners feeling like they are having obligation or service sex, which continues to build resentment and emotional distance.

For Connie and Jay, this stage manifested in their misaligned expectations around intimacy. Jay sought physical intimacy as validation of Connie's love, while Connie needed validation by having an emotional connection with Jay before feeling ready for sex. Their inability to communicate these needs clearly led to hurt feelings on both sides.

As they worked through their issues with me, Connie and Jay began to recognize this pattern in their relationship. They realized that their sexual encounters had often been tinged with anxiety—each wondering if they were truly desired and loved by the other. This realization was both painful and liberating, as it allowed them to see how true intimacy required moving beyond sex as a way to seek reassurance or test the relationship.

## Stage 3: Passionate Intimacy: The Fire that Deepens Connection

Passionate intimacy is the spark that transforms a relationship from ordinary to extraordinary. It's an all-encompassing connection between two partners, intertwining emotional, physical, and even spiritual dimensions. Unlike simple affection or physical intimacy, passionate intimacy goes deeper, fueling a couple's bond and creating a thriving, dynamic partnership.

At its core, passionate intimacy is about vulnerability and authenticity. It requires partners to open themselves fully to one another, sharing their deepest hopes, fears, and desires without reservation. This level of openness can be frightening at first, but it's through this mutual unveiling that true intimacy blossoms.

When two people create passionate intimacy, they experience a heightened awareness of each other. Small gestures take on new meaning—a light touch on the shoulder, catching your partner's eye across a crowded room. There's an almost electric energy between the pair, a magnetic pull drawing them together.

This magnetism shows up in their physical relationship as well, enhancing pleasure and deepening sensations. Sex becomes more than just a physical act. Rather, there is a merging of the physical body, emotions, and energy. Even simple everyday moments—cooking dinner together, taking a walk, or sitting with each other in silence—are infused with tenderness and desire.

Passionate intimacy creates a profound sense of emotional safety and acceptance. Partners become each other's safe haven where they can be fully themselves without fear of judgment. This emotional security allows for greater risk-taking and growth, both individually and as a couple.

Couples are often surprised when they experience the spiritual dimension of passionate intimacy. Many describe it as a feeling of oneness, a blending of energies that goes beyond the physical world. This soul connection can bring a sense of purpose and meaning to the relationship, transforming it into a more powerful and transcendent relationship.

Achieving passionate intimacy requires a focused and persistent effort from both partners, as well as a willingness to explore your own relationship patterns and unresolved trauma and childhood wounds. It blossoms through honest and open communication and a fearless embrace of vulnerability. You must consciously and consistently choose to turn towards each other, even in the face of conflict or stress, while also learning the necessary tools to repair cracks in your relationship bond.

Passionate intimacy also requires a deeper connection on the physical level. While emotional intimacy can exist without physical touch, the power of skin-to-skin contact cannot be underestimated. Partners who cultivate passionate intimacy engage in regular, nonsexual physical touch—holding hands, cuddling, giving massages—to maintain their connection. They also prioritize their sexual relationship, exploring new ways to please each other and keep the spark of desire alive.

This level of intimacy doesn't happen overnight. It's a journey that unfolds over time, requiring patience, commitment, and a willingness to grow together. By reading this book, learning new skills, and completing the exercises, you are taking a huge leap towards creating a lifetime of passionate intimacy.

# 4

# HEALING PAST CHILDHOOD AND RELATIONSHIP WOUNDS

One of the best pieces of advice I've ever received about working with couples is recognizing that the two people sitting in front of me are not two adults, but rather two wounded children. This helps me more quickly attune to them, recognize the emotional wounds they bring to the relationship, and empathize with the pain they both feel.

I'm well aware that many people do not enjoy dredging up painful childhood memories. In fact, I've had some clients get angry with me when I ask about their childhood. For many of us, our childhood memories are in the distant past and should not continue to have control over our lives. Unfortunately, that's not how childhood wounds work.

There's also not a single person on this earth, no matter how "happy" or "normal" their childhood was, who leaves this period of their life unscarred. While the amount and intensity of emotional wounding will vary from person to person, we all carry some childhood wounds that impact our adult intimate relationships. Acknowledging your own emotional wounds, as well as those of your partner, and understanding how they manifest in your relationship is an essential step to creating passionate intimacy.

**Case Study: Carolyn and Ted**

Meet Carolyn and Ted, a Chicago powerhouse couple in their mid-forties who had been married for thirteen years. For the past few years, their physical intimacy had been nonexistent. Carolyn believes that Ted is no longer attracted to her, while Ted feels like he can't do anything right and has stopped trying.

During the course of one of our sessions, Carolyn shared a bit about her childhood. "My family was completely dysfunctional. My Dad was an alcoholic and left when I was seven, and my mom worked two jobs. I was basically a latchkey kid at the age of nine, taking care of me and my younger brother." I gently probed further, asking Carolyn how she felt during those times.

"Alone," she said, her voice barely above a whisper. "I felt so alone and scared all the time, but I had to be strong for my brother."

I leaned forward and said, "You learned pretty early on in life that the only one who you could depend on was yourself. I imagine it's very hard for anyone to be able to meet your needs." Carolyn nodded her head imperceptibly.

I turned to Ted, "And what about you, Ted? What was your childhood like?"

Ted shifted uncomfortably in his seat. "Well, compared to Carolyn's, mine seems pretty normal. I mean, my parents were together, we had enough money..."

"But?" I prompted, sensing there was more.

"My parents were perfectionists. Nothing I did was ever good enough."

I nodded, encouraging Ted to continue. He took a deep breath. "I remember bringing home a report card with all A's except for one B+. Instead of praise, my father asked why the B+ wasn't an A. That's just how it always was. He was always so critical of me. I could never do anything right."

"Ted, all that criticism that you received as a child has caused you to lose confidence in your abilities as a lover."

He nodded in agreement, "I feel like there's nothing I can do right with Carolyn."

I looked at both Carolyn and Ted, seeing the pain in their eyes as they revisited these childhood memories. "What I'm hearing," I said gently, "is that both of you developed coping mechanisms as children that are now affecting your relationship as adults."

Carolyn's brow furrowed. "What do you mean?"

"Carolyn, you learned to be fiercely independent and self-reliant. You had to be. But that means you struggle with vulnerability and allowing others, including Ted, to meet your needs." I turned to Ted. "And you, Ted, internalized all that criticism. It's made you hesitant to take initiative or express yourself freely for fear of doing something wrong."

They both sat silently, absorbing this information. I could see the wheels turning in their minds.

"So how does this play out in your relationship?" I asked.

Carolyn spoke first, her voice trembling slightly. "I...I guess I do have a hard time letting Ted in. I'm always trying to do everything myself, even when I'm exhausted. And when he tries to help, I often brush him off or criticize how he does things."

Ted nodded, a look of realization dawning on his face. "And I've stopped trying to initiate sex because I'm afraid of being rejected or doing something wrong. I feel like I can't meet Carolyn's standards, so why even try?"

I leaned forward, my voice gentle but firm. "This is exactly how your childhood wounds are manifesting in your relationship. Carolyn, your fear of abandonment and need for control is pushing Ted away. And Ted, your fear of criticism is causing you to withdraw, which only reinforces Carolyn's belief that she has to do everything herself."

I watched as understanding dawned on their faces. Carolyn reached out and took Ted's hand, a gesture I hadn't seen from them before.

Over the next few sessions, we worked on exercises to help Carolyn practice vulnerability and allowing Ted to support her. For Ted, we focused on building his confidence and helping him learn to communicate his needs without fear of criticism.

## WHAT IS AN EMOTIONAL WOUND?

An emotional wound is a negative experience (or set of experiences) that causes pain on a deep psychological level. It is a lasting hurt that often involves someone close: a family member, lover, mentor, friend, or other trusted individual. Emotional wounds derive from childhood experiences that cause feelings of fear, rejection, shame, guilt, betrayal, unworthiness, and abandonment, to name a few. Unlike adults, children do not have the emotional or mental capacity to process these experiences, nor do they understand the context in which they occur.

But when these situations occur, the feelings that you went through are stored in your physical body. These stored emotions can later manifest as physical symptoms, behavioral patterns, or emotional reactions that seem disproportionate to the current situation. For Carolyn and Ted, their childhood wounds were clearly influencing their adult relationship dynamics, as is the case for all couples during a conflict.

Lise Bourbeau, a Canadian psychotherapist, is credited with identifying five universal core emotional wounds, each of which occurs at different stages of early childhood development. These wounds frequently surface in adult intimate relationships. It's also not uncommon for someone to have experienced multiple wounds throughout their life, which interact with each other as well.

## REJECTION:

Rejection is the first wound a child feels, and it can also occur in utero if for example you were the result of an unplanned or unwanted pregnancy. The rejection wound happens when a child feels rejected or abandoned. However, it’s important to understand that this is from the perspective of an infant, so even the seemingly innocent decision to put a baby in its own room, separate from their primary caregiver (which until the last few decades was standard practice), can create a rejection wound. If you grew up feeling different from others (if you were the outsider in the family or otherwise on the margins), or if you were someone who was criticized for being neurodiverse, you most likely will have a rejection wound. This wound can make you feel undeserving of love and attention, undesirable, and unworthy.

Experiencing rejection can damage your self-esteem, making it difficult to handle inevitable instances of rejection in later life. It also results in struggles with setting healthy boundaries and taking risks since the fear of failure looms large. Adults with rejection wounds often become perfectionists, withdraw from others, and have an avoidant attachment style which makes it challenging to maintain intimate relationships.

## Abandonment:

The abandonment wound occurs during the ages of one to three. It can manifest in a variety of ways. For myself, the death of my father when I was three years old and my mother's subsequent nervous breakdown caused a deep feeling of loneliness and a constant fear that I could not depend on people I loved to not leave me. My fear of being alone is what kept me in a loveless and sexless marriage for over twenty-six years. It also prevented me from opening myself up to other relationships for fear of that person also abandoning me. Abandonment wounds can also occur from a parent being emotionally disconnected or emotionally distant from a child.

Being abandoned can lead to two extremes: becoming overly reliant on others or fiercely independent. Just like Carolyn, who learned that her needs would never be met by anyone else, one may develop a strong sense of self-sufficiency. People who have experienced abandonment in the past may also unconsciously sabotage their own romantic relationships and even end them themselves to avoid the pain of being abandoned again.

Alternatively, many individuals with abandonment wounds can become extremely needy, end up in codependent relationships, and tend to be anxiously attached, smothering others with their neediness.

## Humiliation:

The humiliation wound occurs during the ages of eighteen months to three years. It results from a child being shamed or degraded by a parent, often in public. At this age, a child can begin to process negative or demeaning comments from adults about their behavior. For example, a toddler who is "caught" touching their private parts and is then told that they are bad or dirty will likely end up with a humiliation wound.

Adults with humiliation wounds tend to be people pleasers, putting others' needs above their own, even to their own detriment. They may have difficulty embracing their own sexuality and finding pleasure because they fear being ridiculed and shamed. Coping with these wounds can lead to a reliance on food as a source of emotional comfort, often resulting in struggles with weight. They also may have feelings of unworthiness and self-disgust or self-loathing.

Some percentage of individuals with this wound may become selfish and tyrannical and frequently humiliate others as a defense mechanism relating to their own sense of humiliation. A perfect example of this is the schoolyard bully who was often humiliated as a child.

## Betrayal:

Between the ages of two to four, children can understand and feel disappointed when a parent does not fulfill a promise, lies to them, or manipulates them. This experience causes them to have significant trust issues. Individuals with a betrayal wound are very controlling, tend not to trust others, and try to impose their will and point of view.

As adults they seek out leadership positions, need to feel special to cover up their own self-worth wounds, can lie and be manipulative to get their way, are often inflexible, are detail oriented, and tend to be planners with multiple checklists. Vulnerability is very challenging for them since they struggle with trust issues and do not feel safe opening up to others. Since the betrayal wound is usually incurred by the parent of the opposite sex of the child, these individuals also have problems trusting their romantic partners.

## Injustice Wound:

The injustice wound occurs during the ages of four to six and results from parents being overly critical, demanding, and authoritarian.

This is a crucial time for a child's development of individuality and autonomy. The criticism they experience makes them feel unworthy or inadequate. As a result of the criticism, they become rigid and strive for perfection, closing off their feelings and emotions.

Individuals who experience injustice wounds rely on facts over feelings and often boast about their knowledge. They will do anything to not show their anger and lose control, and they can appear insensitive and cold and be very critical of others. They also have a tendency to overexert themselves and not respect their own limits (characteristics of type A personalities) and often struggle with intimate relationships due to their challenges with being vulnerable.

### *Childhood Wound Exercise*

1. Looking at your childhood, which of these wounds do you most identify with?
Remember these are universal and we all have experienced each of them at some point, but typically only one or two dominate our behavior.
2. How does that wound show up for you in your life?
3. How does that wound show up for you in your romantic relationship?
4. Identify one or two behaviors that you'd like to change and outline some steps that you might take to implement those changes.

## Healing Your Emotional Wounds

Emotional wounds occur at an early age; thus they become deeply ingrained in our psyches and our behaviors, making it nearly impossible to ever completely erase their impact. However, there are steps you can take to mitigate their effects on your adult relationships.

1. Awareness:

Acknowledging and accepting the wound is the first step towards healing. This involves revisiting childhood memories, which can be painful but is necessary for change to occur.

2. Compassion:

It's important to be kind to yourself and practice self-compassion. Remember that you were just a child when these wounds occurred and had no control over them. The behaviors and defense mechanisms that you developed were important strategies to keep you safe.

3. Share vulnerably with your partner:

Communicate openly about your childhood wounds and the impact they had on you. This can help deepen your relationship and intimacy. Sharing traumatic childhood events with a partner can be challenging, and you'd be surprised at the number of couples who only share their childhood traumas and experiences for the first time during our coaching sessions. Often there's a lot of shame associated with these past experiences, and clients are reluctant to dredge up painful memories. However, being vulnerable and sharing your experiences can help your partner to understand how your childhood has shaped you and allow them to better empathize with you.

4. Seek professional help:

Work with a coach or therapist who specializes in inner child work to learn how to re-parent your inner child. Coaches trained in the Somatica method are an excellent resource for healing childhood wounds. Ultimately this will allow you to develop new and healthier strategies for dealing with your emotional wounds.

Let's take a look at how this new awareness evolved for Ted and Carolyn when I asked them this question: "How might your emotional wounds be affecting your relationship?"

Carolyn realized that her abandonment wound had caused her to build walls around herself, pushing Ted away even as she craved closeness. "I'm always waiting for the other shoe to drop," she admitted. "I keep Ted at arm's length because I'm terrified he'll leave me like my dad did."

Ted nodded in understanding. "And my injustice wound makes me hyper-sensitive to criticism. When Carolyn pushes me away or corrects how I do things, I immediately shut down. I feel like that little boy again, never able to meet impossible standards."

They looked at each other with newfound empathy. For the first time, they could see beyond their surface conflicts to the wounded children within.

## HEALING RELATIONSHIP WOUNDS:

When I start working with a couple, one of the first things I examine is their relationship dynamics. All couples have recognizable patterns which quickly reveal themselves when they enter my office and begin to experience conflict, which is guaranteed to happen every time.

These patterns encompass their coping strategies for dealing with their emotional wounds as well as their attachment styles.

**Attachment Wounds:**

Our desire for intimacy with another human being is a basic human need. We are born completely helpless, "little blobs of protoplasm" as my ex-husband fondly called our infant sons. Without human support to meet our needs for food and shelter, we would quickly die. But infants need more than food and shelter to thrive: They need a strong attachment with a primary caregiver. This attachment sets up key conditions that allow for healthy intimate relationships. Likewise, a lack of attachment predisposes us to encounter difficulty in these crucial areas of our lives.

Attachment theory (which was devised in research by developmental psychologist John Bowlby in the 1960s and 1970s) tells us that children will have different patterns of attachment depending primarily on how they experience their early caregiving environment. Early patterns of attachment shape, but do not determine, the individual's expectations in later relationships.

Attachment theory identifies four distinct attachment styles. According to Bowlby, a child's attachment style results from the caregiver's behavior. It is essentially the way any individual child responds to the adult they interact with the most.

| Attachment Styles | % of sample (also generalized to represent US population) | The child's general state of being | Mother's responsiveness to her child's signals and needs | Fulfillment of the child's needs (why the child acts the way it does) |
|---|---|---|---|---|
| Secure Attachment | 65% | Secure, explorative, happy | Quick, sensitive, consistent | Believes and trusts that his/her needs will be met |
| Avoidant Attachment | 20% | Not very explorative, emotionally distant | Distant, disengaged | Subconsciously believes that his/her needs probably won't be met |
| Ambivalent Attachment | 10-15% | Anxious, insecure, angry | Inconsistent; sometimes sensitive, sometimes neglectful | Cannot rely on his/her needs being met |
| Anxious Avoidant Attachment | 10-15% | Depressed, angry, completely passive, nonresponsive | Extreme, erratic, Frightened or frightening, passive or intrusive | Severely confused with no strategy to have his/her needs met |

Securely attached children: Caregiver responds to child's needs, reacts quickly and positively

Anxiously attached children: Caregiver responds to child's needs inconsistently

Avoidantly attached children: Caregiver is unresponsive, uncaring, dismissive

Anxious avoidant or disorganized attachment: Caregiver is abusive or neglectful, responds in frightening ways.

These attachment styles follow us into our adult life. In their groundbreaking book *Attached* (Tarcher/Penguin 2010), authors Amir Levine and Rachel Heller explain the science of adult attachment and how it impacts our ability to form healthy relationships.

According to Levine and Heller, *"Secure people feel comfortable with intimacy and are usually warm and loving, anxious people crave intimacy, are often preoccupied with their relationships, and tend to worry about their partner's ability to love them back, and avoidant people equate intimacy with a loss of independence and constantly try to minimize closeness."*

Adult attachment styles impact:

- our view of intimacy and togetherness
- the way we deal with conflicts
- our attitude toward sex
- our ability to communicate our wishes and needs
- the expectations we have of our partner and our overall relationship pattern

Before I go into more detail about the four attachment styles, there are a few important caveats as you begin to self-identify your own.

First, attachment wounds can occur from a variety of circumstances that are not necessarily related to the initial attachment with the primary caregiver. For example, a divorce, a separation or the death of a parent can create an attachment wound later in a child's life, even if they were securely attached as an infant.

Second, attachment styles can change over time. In Jessica Fern's book *Polysecure*, she talks about the concept of "earned secure attachment," which happens over time through growth and personal development, transforming an insecure attachment style into a more secure one.

Third, attachment styles occur on a spectrum and will vary depending on the attachment style of your partner. For example, although I am mostly anxiously attached, when I was with a man who had a strong anxious attachment wound and suffocated me with his need for constant reassurance, my avoidant tendencies took over.

While most coaches and therapists will place individuals in one of the four categories (secure, anxious, avoidant, disorganized), I prefer to use a two-dimensional scale which has recently been embraced by attachment researchers. This scale includes attachment anxiety and attachment avoidance and places individuals in one of four quadrants. One of the benefits of using this scale is that you can place yourself anywhere within a quadrant, which allows context to be taken into consideration.

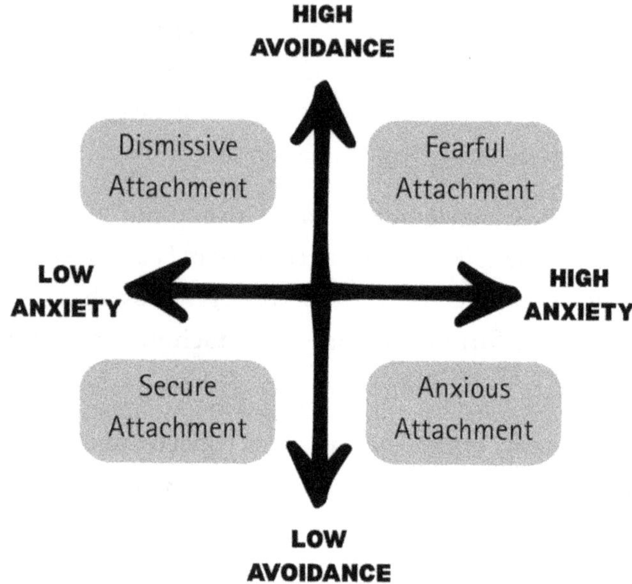


Secure Attachment: If you are low in anxiety and low in avoidance, you fall within the secure attachment style.

Preoccupied: If you are high in anxiety and low in avoidance, you fall within the preoccupied attachment style, also known as "anxious attachment."

Dismissive: If you are low in anxiety and high in avoidance, you fall within the dismissive attachment style, also known as "avoidant attachment."

Fearful: If you are both high in anxiety and high in avoidance, you fall within the fearful-avoidant attachment style, also known as "disorganized."

This scale allows one to better understand how you can transition from an anxious or avoidant attachment style to one that is more secure.

As an example, if you find yourself in the preoccupied quadrant but you are able to utilize techniques to overcome your fear of abandonment by your partner, over time your anxiety will decrease, and you will move closer towards a more secure attachment style.

## THE PURSUER-DISTANCER CYCLE

While every intimate relationship has its own dynamic, there are some common relationship patterns that occur. The most prevalent one (which some estimate shows up over 80 percent of the time) is the pursuer-distancer cycle identified by the renowned couples therapist John Gottman, who aptly named it the "pursuer-distancer dance."

This is by far the most common relationship pattern, because each of us tends to attract into our life people with character traits that we have unconsciously disowned. The pursuer craves intimacy and is unaware of their need for autonomy. The distancer craves autonomy and is unaware of their need for intimacy. In reality, we all crave both intimacy and independence. Partners in healthy relationships learn to find a balance between fulfilling their own individual needs while also meeting the needs of their significant other for connection and personal space.

This is how the pursuer-distancer cycle works. The pursuer, with the more anxious attachment style, wants attention, closeness, and affection in the relationship with their partner. They enjoy talking about their day and sharing their feelings, and they feel a strong sense of rejection when their partner requires space. This may cause the pursuer to criticize their partner and voice complaints in order to meet their need for deeper connection and reassurance. Unfortunately, the pursuer's behavior further alienates the distancer, which in turn triggers the pursuer's abandonment fears and causes them to pursue even more intensely.

Distancers, with their more avoidant attachment style, require emotional distance and physical space when they are under stress. They value independence and autonomy and enjoy spending time alone. They can easily become overwhelmed by the pursuer's neediness and have a low tolerance for conflict. As a result, they will spend more time turning inward or engaging in outside activities, distancing themselves even further from the pursuer.

If this pattern is not interrupted, it will lead to built-up resentment, ultimately creating a toxic contemptuous relationship that cannot be sustained. In fact, Gottman has correctly predicted that failure to transform the distancer-pursuer cycle is one of the key markers of a relationship heading to divorce.

## The Somatic Approach to Sex and Intimacy

One of the ways in which my coaching differs from traditional talk therapy is that I proudly use an experiential, somatic based approach that I learned through extensive training with the Somatica® Institute, cofounded in 2011 by my mentors and teachers, the brilliant Dr. Danielle Harel and Celeste Hirschman, MA. Harel and Hirschman created the Somatica Method®, a unique and powerful embodied approach to sex and intimacy which they developed over twenty years of working in the field with clients. Rather than talking to clients about their sex life, this approach provides clients with a felt sense of intimacy, desire, and eroticism. As I like to tell my clients, "You can't talk your way into a better sex life, you have to feel your way into it."

The Somatica Institute is widely recognized by certifying organizations in the field, and founders Danielle Harel and Celeste Hirschman have created an extensive body of work and resources published on their website and in their three books, many of which I refer to in this book, and have trained over fifteen hundred certified Somatica sex and intimacy coaches throughout the United States and the world. (See the Resources section at the end of the book to link to their directory of certified practitioners.) The Somatica Method is now receiving worldwide recognition through *Virgin Island;*, this award winning reality TV show, produced by UK Channel 4, has captured the hearts and minds of British young adults and brought healing and hope to the sexually inexperienced. The show follows twelve young adults as they are coached by Hirschman and Harel, the lead sexologists on the show, to overcome blocks to sex and intimacy.

While working with my clients Carolyn and Ted, I used the Somatica method to allow them to experience the nuances of the pursuer-distancer cycle in their body.

“Let’s play a game,” I said. “Carolyn, you go to one corner of the room, and Ted, you go to the other. Now each of you are going to take turns moving a few steps towards each other.”

Carolyn and Ted looked at each other uncertainly but followed my instructions. They stood in opposite corners of my office, facing each other.

“All right, Carolyn, you go first,” I said. “Take a few steps towards Ted.”

Carolyn hesitated for a moment, then slowly walked three steps towards her husband. Ted tensed visibly as she approached.

“Now Ted, it's your turn. Take a few steps towards Carolyn.”

Ted took two small steps forward, keeping his arms crossed over his chest.

“Good,” I said. “Now Carolyn, move towards Ted again.”

This time, Carolyn moved more quickly, taking four large strides that brought her quite close to Ted. He immediately took a step back.

“Interesting,” I noted. “Ted, why did you step back?”

“I... I don't know,” Ted stammered. “It just felt like she was coming towards me really fast, and I needed more space.”

“Carolyn, how did that make you feel when Ted took a step back”, I gently probed.

“I felt like he was rejecting me. I wanted to be closer to him.”

I smiled. “This is exactly what happens in the distancer-pursuer cycle. Carolyn, as the pursuer, you move towards Ted seeking closeness and connection. But Ted, as the distancer, feels overwhelmed by this and retreats, needing more space. This in turn makes you feel rejected, Carolyn, so you pursue him even more intensely. And Ted, feeling pressured, withdraws further. Do you see how this cycle perpetuates itself?”

Both Carolyn and Ted nodded slowly, a look of realization dawning on their faces.

“Let's try something different,” I suggested. “Carolyn, this time when you move towards Ted, I want Ted to put up his hand when he feels you’re getting too close and ask you to take a few steps backward.”

Carolyn and Ted repeated the exercise, and this time, when Carolyn started approaching too fast, Ted put up his hand to stop her.

Carolyn paused and took a few steps backward. They stood facing each other for a minute and when it was Ted’s turn, much to Carolyn’s surprise, he moved towards her.

I smiled, seeing the shift in their dynamic. “Excellent. Now, let's discuss what just happened. Ted, how did it feel to be able to set a boundary?”

Ted's posture had relaxed visibly. “It felt...empowering. Like I had some control over the situation.”

"And Carolyn," I turned to her, "how did it feel to respect Ted's boundary?"

Carolyn thought for a moment. "At first, I felt a bit rejected. But then...I realized Ted wasn't pushing me away completely. He just needed a bit more space."

"Exactly," I nodded. "And what happened next, Ted?"

"I felt more comfortable moving towards Carolyn," Ted admitted. "I didn't feel pressured, so I actually wanted to get closer."

"This is a crucial lesson," I explained. "When the distancer feels they have control over their space and their autonomy is being respected, they often feel more comfortable moving towards connection on their own terms."

Carolyn and Ted looked at each other, a new understanding passing between them.

"So how can we apply this to our daily lives?" Carolyn asked, her voice filled with hope.

I walked towards them slowly, eager to build on their breakthrough. "Great question, Carolyn. The key is to recognize when this cycle is happening and consciously choose to break it. Ted, when you feel overwhelmed and need space, instead of withdrawing silently, try to communicate that need clearly and respectfully to Carolyn."

Ted nodded thoughtfully. "I could say something like, 'I'm feeling a bit overwhelmed right now. Could I have some time to myself, and we can reconnect in an hour?'"

"Exactly," I nodded approvingly. "And Carolyn, when Ted expresses this need, it's important for you to respect it without taking it personally. Remember, it's not about rejection—it's about Ted needing to recharge so he can be more present with you later."

Carolyn took a deep breath. "I can see how that would be helpful. But what about when I'm feeling the need for connection?"

"Great question," I replied. "In those moments, instead of pursuing Ted more intensely, try to express your need directly but gently. You could say something like, 'I'm feeling a bit disconnected right now. When you're ready, I'd love to spend some quality time together.'"

Both Carolyn and Ted nodded, absorbing this new approach.

"The key," I continued, "is to communicate your needs to each other when they arise and actively listen to how your partner responds. Recognize when you're in your pattern and take concrete steps to break it."

Recognizing and tending to your childhood wounds is not about blame—it's about understanding. When you can see your partner not as the enemy, but as someone carrying their own emotional wounds, you create space for compassion and deeper connection. Healing doesn't mean becoming perfect or "fixing" yourself—it means becoming more aware, more present, and more accepting of yourself and your partner. And as you begin to soften your protective defenses and trust each other with your most tender truths, a new language of emotional intimacy begins to emerge.

There is no one-size-fits-all approach to emotional intimacy; we all have our unique way of connecting emotionally with our partner. In the next chapter, we will explore the different ways in which couples connect emotionally, and you will see how learning your partner's unique emotional intimacy language will transform your relationship from surviving to thriving.

# PART TWO
# EMOTIONAL INTIMACY—THE CORE COMPONENT OF PASSIONATE INTIMACY

In this section of the book, we dive into the diverse languages of intimacy, exploring how we give and receive love. You will learn many important skills (attunement, presence, reading body language) to help you better understand your unique way of connecting with your partner. We then focus on vulnerability—the essence of creating connection and intimacy. Finally, we turn to emotional resilience and conflict repair, one of the most important skills a couple needs to master in order to create a healthy long-term relationship.

# 5
# THE DIFFERENT LANGUAGES OF EMOTIONAL INTIMACY

This chapter will take you on a journey to explore the different languages of emotional intimacy and how they can deepen your connection with your partner. Through this exploration, you will discover how you give and receive love, as well as gain insight into expressing your needs and feelings effectively. You will learn to attune yourself to your partner's energy, feeling their emotions and understanding their thoughts without words. And in the moments of intimate silence between you, you will harness a special power that brings you closer together in understanding and communication.

## THE POWER OF PRESENCE IN BUILDING EMOTIONAL INTIMACY

What is your understanding of being present, and how can you tell if you are truly present or not? This is one of the first questions I ask a couple when we begin our work together.

Most of us understand what it's like not to be present: You are scrolling through your phone, and your thoughts are wandering; your physical body is in the room, but your head and heart are someplace else. Being present means that you are fully occupying your body, and you are aware of body sensations and attuned to all five of your senses. Your attention is focused inside, and you have access to your feelings and emotions. You feel grounded and solid and supported by the earth underneath your feet.

It is only when you are truly present with yourself that you have the ability to also be present with your partner. So often I see someone "trying" to be present with their partner, but they are so disconnected from themselves that true presence is impossible.

They may be nodding and saying "mmhmm" at the right moments, but their eyes are glazed over and their energy is scattered. Their partner can sense this disconnection, even if they can't quite put their finger on what feels off.

Meditation and mindfulness practices are excellent ways to learn how to presence. You can also try one of my grounding exercises here. https://www.passionateintimacyretreats.com/go-deeper/ If you need a quick grounding practice, close your eyes, feel your feet on the ground, take a few deep breaths, and feel the rise and fall of your chest. Slowly open your eyes and let your attention settle into the present moment.

Once you feel grounded in your own body, you can begin to establish presence with your partner. Turn towards them and establish eye contact while you continue to breathe and feel your own body connected to the earth. Give your partner your undivided attention and use body language (a nod, or a hand on their arm or leg) to amplify your presence.

## *PRESENCE EXERCISE:*

This powerful exercise will help you recognize what being truly present with your partner feels like. The interesting thing about being present with your partner is that presence truly is in the eyes of the beholder. If your partner tells you they can't feel your presence or that your presence has waned, you have to take their word for it and understand that they are expressing their own perception and experience.

1. Stand at about an arm's-length distance across from your partner. One person will be the Giver and the other will be the Receiver.
2. The Giver closes their eyes, feels their feet on the ground, and establishes presence inwardly.
3. The Giver opens their eyes and tries to be present with the Receiver without using words. The Giver maintains eye contact and presence for as long as they can.
4. The Receiver becomes very aware of the Giver. When the Receiver feels like the Giver has lost some presence, they gently tap the Giver's chest.
5. The Giver takes note of this and tries to re-establish presence, taking a moment if necessary to inwardly ground before reconnecting with the Receiver.
Continue this exercise for 2 to 3 minutes, then debrief.
6. Switch roles so the Receiver becomes the Giver and the Giver becomes the Receiver.

Pitfalls to look out for:

Maintaining presence for several minutes is very challenging for most people, so be kind to yourself. It gets easier the more you practice mindfulness.

Receivers tend to confer the benefit of the doubt on Givers. Don't give in to this temptation. If you feel like your partner's energy shifted, if they start looking around the room, tap them on the chest. Presence involves working with subtle energy, so you should respond even to subtle changes you notice in your partner.

This is not a staring contest, but we do send out many signals and energy just with our eyes. If the eye gazing feels too intense for either one of you, take a break, close your eyes, and see if you can both come back into the exercise.

Givers, although I do not want you to ever argue with your partner when they tap you on the chest indicating they were not feeling your presence, it is important for you to notice inside of your body what might have shifted when this happens. Were you in your head for a moment, did you lose the feeling of your feet on the ground, did your eyes wander?

**Attunement:**

A key component of emotional intimacy is being able to attune to your partner, which is impossible if you are not present. Attunement is a deep form of listening and understanding that goes beyond just hearing words. It involves tuning into your partner's emotional state, body language, and energy. When you're attuned to your partner, you can sense their mood shifts, pick up on subtle cues, and respond empathetically to their needs.

When you are well attuned to your partner, you are like two tuning forks. When you strike a tuning fork and set it to vibrating, a second tuning fork set at the same pitch will begin to vibrate with the first fork, emitting the same pleasant vibrational sound. Conversely, when you are misaligned, the two tuning forks are set to different pitches, creating a dissonant sound. This lack of attunement can lead to misunderstandings, hurt feelings, and a sense of disconnection.

Some signals that you and partner are not attuned include:

- Feeling like you are out of synch with each other
- Comments like "You don't get me" or "You never really listen to me"
- Feeling emotionally distant even when you're physically close
- Unable to move rhythmically with each other
- Initiating or having sex feels awkward and may end up in conflict

### *ATTUNEMENT EXERCISE:*

1. Sit facing each other, maintaining comfortable eye contact.
2. Take a few deep breaths together, synchronizing your breathing. As you will learn later in the book, breathing together is one of the most powerful ways to attune to and connect with your partner's energy.
3. One partner (the Sender) thinks of a specific emotion or memory that evokes strong feelings without expressing it verbally or through obvious facial expressions.
4. The other partner (the Receiver) tries to sense and name the emotion, while observing the Sender's facial expressions, body language and energy.
5. After a minute, the Receiver shares what they sensed about the Sender's emotional state.
6. The Sender then reveals what they were feeling or thinking about.
7. Take a few minutes to discuss how accurate the Receiver's perception was and what cues they noticed.
8. Switch roles and repeat.

Practice this exercise regularly, and you'll find your ability to attune to each other improving over time.

**Learn How to Read Body Language**

Communication between partners happens on so many different levels; verbal, nonverbal, and energetic. Nonverbal communication, however, is one of the most powerful forms of communication in intimate relationships. Your body is constantly sending signals about your emotional state, even when you're not aware of it. Learning to read your partner's body language can significantly enhance your emotional connection.

When learning to read body language, pay close attention to the following:

1. Eye contact—Notice if your partner is looking at you directly or looking away. There is a saying that the eyes are the windows to the soul and it is true, you can often see what someone is feeling by looking into their eyes.

2. Facial expressions—The face is incredibly expressive. Notice whether your partner is smiling, frowning, raising their eyebrows or furrowing them.

3. Posture—Notice how your partner holds their body. Are their arms crossed, are their hands clasped, do they appear tense and contracted or open and relaxed?

4. Gestures—-Hand gestures, a tilt of the head, or a roll of the eyes can convey a wealth of information.

Very often your partner might be saying one thing to you while their body language says something completely different. This is one of the major stumbling blocks to creating emotional intimacy. For example, imagine that you're asking your partner if they are upset that you didn't want to have sex last night. They might say, "No, it's totally fine," but their crossed arms, tense shoulders, and averted gaze tell a totally different story. In these cases, it's important to gently point out the discrepancy you're noticing. "You say you're not upset, but you won't look at me and your shoulders seem tense. Do you want to talk about it?"

This level of communication provides an opening for a conversation about each of your feelings, prevents resentment from building up, and allows you to quickly repair a tiny fissure in the relationship.

### *Exercise: The Mirror Game*

This exercise will help you become more aware of your partner's body language and nonverbal cues.

1. Stand facing each other about arm's length apart.
2. One partner (the Leader) begins to move slowly, making various gestures and facial expressions.
3. The other partner (the Follower) tries to mirror these movements and expressions as closely as possible, as if they were the Leader's reflection in a mirror.
4. After a few minutes, switch roles.
5. Repeat the exercise, but this time, the Leader should incorporate emotions into their movements and expressions. For example, they might act out feeling sad, angry, or excited.
6. Discuss your experience afterward. What was easy or challenging about mirroring your partner? Did you notice any habitual gestures or expressions your partner uses?

This exercise not only helps you become more attuned to your partner's nonverbal cues but also promotes empathy and connection. By physically embodying your partner's movements and expressions, you gain insight into how they somatically express their emotional state.

## The Language of Touch

Later in this book, we will spend a significant amount of time talking about the importance of touch in strengthening your physical relationship and intimacy. However, touch is a very powerful form of nonverbal communication that can also convey a vast array of emotional states.

Touch is the first of your senses that develops in utero, and as such, is the first language that you learn. Soft, gentle touch releases oxytocin into the bloodstream, creating a feeling of warmth and trust with your partner.

Touch is one of the most powerful tools we have for emotional connection and communication in your relationship. The way you touch your partner can convey comfort, reassurance, desire, playfulness, frustration, or even anger.

When I'm working with a couple, I'm always both tracking their body language and noticing how much or little they touch each other during the session. This helps me assess what their individual emotional states are and how they are feeling about each other and the relationship. When they begin to reconnect, I will frequently see one partner reach out for the other's hand or leg. When their bodies are actually touching on the sofa, I immediately know that they are feeling safe and connected with each other.

## Hugging Creates Connection

How often do you hug your partner? Once a day, a week, a month? What does that hug convey to you? Is it deep and long, or is it short and perfunctory?

Most couples do not know how to hug in a way that creates emotional connection and closeness. I know this for a fact because I always ask couples to show me how they hug each other. The hug is generally very short, often without even their full bodies touching. This may be how you hug your relatives, but it is definitely not how you should hug your intimate partner.

Learning to give a proper, heartfelt hug can be transformative for your relationship. A deep, intentional hug releases oxytocin, reduces stress, and fosters a sense of safety and connection.

### *Exercise: Heart to Heart Melting Hug*

1. Stand facing each other and establish eye contact.
2. Take a few deep breaths together to ground yourself.
3. Slowly move in for the hug, making sure that the front of each of your bodies makes full contact with your partner. Wrap your arms around each other, finding a comfortable position.
4. Feel your bellies touching and take five deep, slow breaths together.
5. Allow yourself to fully relax into your partner's body and arms. The image I like to use is that you are like a pat of butter melting into the pan.
6. Notice if you can let go even further, melting your bodies and your hearts together.
7. Maintain the hug for as long as you can, but at least for one minute. Generally, when I coach my clients through this exercise, they hug for between three to five minutes.

Take just five minutes a day to embrace in a melting hug, and you'll be amazed at the increase in emotional connection between you and your partner.

## THE POWER OF SILENCE

It's taken me a long time to recognize that being in silence with your partner is actually a way to deepen your emotional connection. For decades, my ex-husband and I would sit in silence when we were out to dinner, after exhausting all conversation about mundane matters. That silence felt like a huge abyss between us since there was absolutely no emotional intimacy or connection in our relationship. It was torturous for me to look around a restaurant and see couples smiling and talking with each other, clearly enjoying being in each other's company. In fact, the moment I made the decision to leave my marriage was during our 25th anniversary dinner, where we sat in a complete silence filled with contempt.

Until recently, being in silence was a big trigger for me and I would often feel anxious and compelled to fill the quiet with chatter. However, as I've grown in my own emotional awareness and Daren and I have deepened our intimacy, I've come to appreciate the power of comfortable silence with a partner.

Silence can be a profound form of communication when you're truly emotionally connected with a partner. It's a safe space where you can simply be together, attuned to and present with each other without the need for words. This kind of silence is rich with meaning and intimacy.

Some of the most emotionally intimate moments in a relationship happen in silence; lying in bed resting on each other after making love, holding hands while out on a walk, and sitting on the couch and cuddling. These silent moments allow for a deep, wordless bonding where you feel completely in sync with each other and experience a connection more powerful than any conversation.

This type of silence is very different from the awkward or tense silences that occur when there's disconnection or conflict in a relationship. Those silences feel heavy and uncomfortable, whereas comfortable silence feels light, peaceful, and connecting.

Learning to be comfortable with silence in your relationship can greatly enhance your emotional intimacy. It allows you to practice being present with each other, attune to each other's energy and emotions, and synchronize your nervous systems.

### *Silent Connection Exercise:*

1. Sit facing each other, close enough that your knees are almost touching.
2. Set a timer for five minutes (you can gradually increase this time as you become more comfortable).
3. Make eye contact with your partner. If direct eye contact feels uncomfortable, you can try softening your eyes and shift your gaze more towards your partner's forehead.
4. Take a few deep breaths together to ground yourselves.
5. For the duration of the timer, simply sit in silence together. Don't speak or try to communicate in any way. Just be present with each other.
6. Notice what you're feeling in your body. Are you tense or relaxed? What sensations do you notice?
7. Observe your partner. What do you notice about their facial expressions, their breathing, their energy?
8. If your mind wanders, gently bring your attention back to the present moment and your partner.
9. When the timer goes off, take a moment to slowly come out of the exercise.
10. Discuss your experience with each other. What did you notice? How did it feel to be in silence together?

This exercise might feel uncomfortable at first, especially if you're not used to prolonged eye contact or sitting in silence with your partner. Eye contact can sometimes feel extremely vulnerable. It's a very intimate way of connecting with your partner. However, as you continue to do this exercise, over time, you'll notice that you will be able to relax more and start enjoying these silent moments with your partner.

## THE FIVE LOVE LANGUAGES

Understanding how you like to give and receive love is an important step towards creating passionate intimacy. The concept of the five love languages was created by Dr. Gary Chapman, a renowned counselor and author. He codified his work in the *New York Times* best-selling book, *The 5 Love Languages: The Secret to Love That Lasts* (1992). Chapman based his groundbreaking concept on the work that he did with thousands of couples, who despite believing that they were showing love to each other, still felt emotionally disconnected and misunderstood.

Chapman identified five different styles of expressing love and created a simple test to help individuals to determine what their love languages are in order of priority. I have all my couples take this test, and I highly recommend that you and your partner take it as well: https://5lovelanguages.com/quizzes/love-language

### 1. WORDS OF AFFIRMATION

If words of affirmation are your love language, then it's important for you to receive acknowledgment, compliments, and other forms of spoken appreciation from your partner so that you feel seen, valued, and cherished. During sex, you may also desire your partner to be very verbal, telling you how "hot," beautiful, or special you are.

Beyond the bedroom, hearing "I love you" frequently, receiving text messages filled with kind words, or even being told how much your presence is appreciated after a long day can fill your emotional tank. These verbal affirmations are like oxygen for someone whose primary love language is words of affirmation; without them, you may feel unloved or taken for granted.

## 2. Acts of Service

Individuals with acts of service as their love language receive love best when their partner does errands for them, takes care of the laundry, washes their car, and so on. In this case, actions do speak louder than words. Being considered and taken care of makes you special and loved.

During sex, you may want your partner to ensure the room is set up just right, perhaps with dim lighting and sexy music. You might appreciate them taking the time to prepare everything beforehand. You may also want them to put your pleasure first and make sure you're comfortable and satisfied. Showing this level of thoughtfulness and consideration makes you feel truly cared for and loved.

## 3. Spending Quality Time

If quality time is your love language, then it's all about the experience of having the undivided attention of your partner. Deep emotional conversations and spending hours in intimate connection are essential. It's during these interactions that you feel most connected and valued as they provide the opportunity for genuine companionship and bonding. Without this dedicated time together, you may feel neglected or distant.

Quickies are probably not your thing. You'd rather spend time staring into your partner's eyes, sharing feelings, taking a leisurely bath together, and slowly moving towards sensual touch. These activities not only allow you to enjoy each other's presence but also build a strong emotional bond. The gradual build-up of connection through meaningful interactions makes every touch and gesture more significant.

## 4. Physical Touch:

Consistent embodied connection is important if your love language is physical touch. This includes all kinds of touch, including hugs, holding hands, a gentle touch on the arm, and nurturing touch (for example, having your hair stroked while lying in your partner's lap or arms). You may feel rejected if you don't receive touch, leading to emotional distance.

During sex, you desire a lot of sensual touch, light massage, and an array of tactile experiences. You crave the warmth of your partner's skin against yours, the pressure of their hands exploring your body, and the feel of their breath on your neck. Foreplay is the main event for you, and the connection of your bodies is true intimacy with no need for words.

## 5. Receiving Gifts

If receiving gifts is your love language, it's important to understand that it's not about the material aspect but the thoughtfulness and effort behind a gift. The act of giving and receiving gifts becomes a symbol of love and affection. You feel most cherished when your partner surprises you with thoughtful presents, big or small. These gifts serve as tangible reminders of your partner's love and consideration.

In the realm of sex, this love language might manifest as your partner presenting you with sensual gifts like lingerie, massage oils, or even sex toys. The effort put into selecting these items specifically for your pleasure can be deeply satisfying and can make you feel incredibly desired. You might also appreciate romantic gestures like rose petals scattered on the bed or a carefully planned romantic getaway.

It's important to remember that your love languages can change over time, depending on the context and the person with whom you are in a relationship. Also, most people have multiple love languages; the test results will help you identify what your primary ones are. You may have one love language in the bedroom and one for everyday life. You also may have different love languages for giving and receiving love. For example, touch may be the way you want to receive love, but you may give love through acts of service.

When learning about your own and your partner's love languages, it's important to keep an open mind and not be judgmental. No one love language is "better" than another. What's important is being able to identify your love languages. Understand that is not uncommon for your own and your partner's love languages to differ. This need not create conflict in your relationship so long as you both acknowledge the differences and make your best efforts to meet some of each other's needs in giving and receiving love.

In my own relationship, words of appreciation are extremely important for me, especially during sex. This is definitely not my partner's comfort zone. The way he gives love is through acts of service, which is considerably lower on my list. Over time, I've learned to appreciate how his making my special tea every morning is one of his ways of saying he loves me, even though I may not hear words as frequently as I would like during sex. I've learned how to process some of my disappointment (a critical skill that we will talk about in Chapter 8), and how to get some of those needs met outside of the bedroom. Ultimately, the more you understand about and appreciate each other's love languages, the easier it will be to create a deep emotional connection and passionate intimacy.

## *Love Languages Exercise*

1. Before taking the test, write down what you think your primary and secondary love language is. Do the same for your partner.
2. Once you receive your results, evaluate whether these languages are the way you both give and receive love. If there is a difference, note that down.
3. Compare your results to your partner's and discuss how this shows up in both your daily life and your sexual relationship.
4. Reflect on past misunderstandings or conflicts in your relationship. Can you identify instances where differences in love languages may have played a role?
5. Create a plan to incorporate each other's love languages into your daily routine. For example, if your partner's primary love language is acts of service, you might commit to doing one thoughtful task for them each day.
6. Explore how your love languages manifest in your sexual relationship. Discuss ways to incorporate each other's love languages into your intimate moments.
7. Practice expressing love in your partner's preferred language, even if it feels unnatural at first. Remember, the goal is to make your partner feel loved and appreciated.
8. Regularly check in with each other about how well you're meeting each other's needs. Be open to feedback and willing to make adjustments.

Learning to speak your partner's language of intimacy isn't just about giving the right kind of touch or saying the right thing—it's about learning to listen differently. Through presence, attunement, and emotional fluency, you begin to understand not just what your partner is saying, but what they're feeling. These exercises aren't meant to perfect your relationship—they're meant to deepen it. When you show up with curiosity, read between the lines, and meet your partner with compassion, you're not just improving your communication—you're strengthening the invisible thread that holds you together.

This next chapter is about the bravest kind of connection. Vulnerability is the secret ingredient that turns communication into true intimacy. Drawing on the work of researchers like Brené Brown, we'll explore how vulnerability disarms shame, builds trust, and becomes the foundation for emotional and sexual intimacy.

# 6
# Vulnerability Is Sexy

There's a shirt that I wear to the gym that always makes people stop and stare for a moment. It says, "Vulnerability is Sexy." For the most part, I get nods and thumbs-ups from women, and men look at me quizzically, confusion all over their faces. This makes total sense since most men are socialized from a very early age to believe that expressing emotions is a sign of weakness.

Spend thirty minutes on a playground and you may see this occur in real time. What happens when a little girl falls down and starts crying? Her parent goes to her, holds her, lets her cry, and comforts her. But when this happens to a little boy, the most common response is to tell him, "Don't cry, you're fine," and send him on his way.

While some of this behavior is thankfully changing in younger generations of parents, those of us born in Generation X or earlier were not so lucky. I frequently hear from my male clients how their fathers were "stoic," did not express emotions, and were not emotionally available to them. There are also other distinct cultural and socioeconomic differences.

I remember a client, Jake, who grew up in a traditional southern family in Alabama.. He recounted how his father never once told him "I love you" or gave him a hug. Any display of affection was considered weak and unmanly. Jake struggled for years with forming deep, meaningful relationships with women because he had never learned how to be emotionally open.

This emotional suppression also exists in communities across various ethnicities and is deeply ingrained in those who serve in the military. "Toughing it out" and not showing signs of "weakness" are expected of men, who are also the providers and protectors, leaving no room for emotional expression other than anger, let alone vulnerability.

While men generally struggle much more with vulnerability due to their socialization, there are plenty of women who also have challenges in this area. This is especially true for women who are fiercely independent and self-sufficient, as they have learned from a young age that adults could not be relied upon for emotional support.

However, without vulnerability, true intimacy is not attainable. As we discussed in Chapter 3, intimacy (in-to-me-see) requires you to reveal your authentic self, with all your imperfections and the battle wounds that shape who you truly are.

Some of my male clients have asked me why vulnerability is so attractive to their female partners. It's a great question, and honestly, I've struggled with coming up with an answer that makes sense to them. Ultimately, I believe that vulnerability happens in our heart space, it makes us feel like our partner is also a human being, who has flaws just like we do. In that way, vulnerability in some way eases our own anxieties about the messiness of both our inner and outer worlds. It also demonstrates a level of emotional intelligence that many women crave, one that is sadly missing in many individuals.

When I asked my partner this question, he had a different take, which I am offering here as well. When a woman senses a man's vulnerability, it reassures her that he has empathy and sensitivity that will likely enable him to not only treat her and others with kindness and compassion but also be a good role model for children.

## THE SCIENCE OF VULNERABILITY

We can't talk about vulnerability without discussing the work of the renowned vulnerability researcher Brené Brown. Brown's groundbreaking research has shed light on the power of vulnerability in fostering connection, creativity, and overall well-being. In her book *Daring Greatly*, she defines vulnerability as "uncertainty, risk, and emotional exposure." It's about showing up and being seen, even when there are no guarantees. One of Brown's key findings is that vulnerability is not a weakness, but rather a strength that can lead to greater intimacy, creativity, and authenticity in our lives.

According to Brown, vulnerability is the birthplace of innovation, creativity, and change. When we allow ourselves to be vulnerable, we open ourselves up to new possibilities and experiences. In the context of romantic relationships, vulnerability helps to deepen connections and provides space for us to challenge some of our false beliefs and misconceptions about intimacy.

I'm going to take a page from my own playbook in *Living an Orgasmic Life* and be completely honest with you about my own struggles with vulnerability. If you've read my previous book, you'll be familiar with the fact that I grew up without any emotional support from my extremely narcissistic mother, who relied on me as her emotional crutch after my father died at age forty-six. Their relationship was highly codependent, and she leaned on me for comfort and stability. That's a lot of pressure to place on a young child, and there was absolutely no room for my emotions, which I did a great job of suppressing for over fifty years.

As a result, I became one of those highly independent, self-sufficient, invulnerable women who has little access to her emotions. In my marriage, I desperately desired closeness with my then-husband but was unable to open up to him. Most of the time I was emotionally numb. Occasionally I would feel some sadness about the state of our sexless and loveless marriage, but then I would go immediately into overwhelm, once again shutting down all my emotions. I struggled to feel empathy for my husband, who like my mother, needed a tremendous amount of emotional support.

It's fair to say that my personal work over the last two decades has been focused on getting more comfortable with vulnerability in both my emotional and sexual expression. By attending dozens of personal growth and sexuality workshops and trainings, as well as working with therapists, coaches, and spiritual guides, I slowly began to chip away at the hard outer shell that protected my heart and my emotions.

My intimate relationships have followed a similar pattern. Each time I chose a partner who slowly allowed me to gradually open up and created some level of emotional safety. It was a less than perfect journey, and I frequently found myself repeating some of my past behaviors, such as choosing narcissistic men as relationship partners.

I've also had the unique opportunity to experience and practice vulnerability through the Somatica® sex and intimacy training program. More than anything, that program pushed me to sit in the discomfort of my vulnerability, sometimes even causing me to experience a significant "shame-over." Named after a hangover, a shame-over occurs when you've exposed more of yourself emotionally than you're comfortable with, leading to feelings of intense vulnerability and shame. These shame-overs were particularly challenging for me, often leaving me feeling raw and exposed for days afterward.

However, each time I pushed through these uncomfortable feelings, I found myself growing stronger and more resilient. These shame-overs were intense but ultimately healing. I learned to sit with the discomfort and the realization that vulnerability, even when it feels excruciating, doesn't kill you. It actually makes you stronger.

One particular exercise in the Somatica program stands out in my memory. We were paired up and asked to take turns sharing something with a partner we were ashamed about. At first, I felt my old defenses rising, as the urge to deflect or minimize my true feelings became almost overwhelming. But as I looked into my partner's eyes, seeing their own vulnerability reflected back at me, I found the courage to open up.

I shared about my experience as a young child allowing my dog Lucky to lick my underwear, which I gently pulled back so he could get his tongue onto my pussy. It was the first time I'd experienced any sexual pleasure, but it was coupled with both anxiety, since I was sure my mother would walk into the room, as well as shame, since I "knew" that this was wrong. This experience created a tremendous amount of stress for me around oral sex, which I could not enjoy until my fifties.

My partner reached out, held my hands, and asked me to look into her eyes, because mine were downcast. As I looked up into my partner's eyes, I expected to see judgment or disgust. Instead, I saw only compassion and acceptance. She squeezed my hands gently and said, "Thank you for sharing that with me. It must have been really difficult to carry that shame for so long."

Her words and the warmth in her eyes broke something open inside me. Suddenly, I was sobbing, years of pent-up shame and guilt pouring out of me. My partner simply held space for me, allowing me to feel everything without trying to fix or change it.

When my tears finally subsided, I felt lighter than I had in years. The shame that had weighed on me for so long began to dissipate, replaced by a sense of relief and even pride in my courage to be vulnerable. This experience was a turning point for me. It showed me the transformative power of vulnerability in a way I had never experienced before.

## Vulnerability Requires Facing Your Shame

In my book, *Living an Orgasmic Life,* I wrote a whole chapter on sexual shame entitled, "Shame: The Nastiest Five Letter Word in the Universe." This chapter delves into the complex topic of sexual shame, exploring its origins and how it is shaped by one's upbringing. Through a multitude of client stories, I demonstrate how individuals have been able to overcome their sexual shame and heal from its effects.

While sexual shame is clearly a barrier to intimacy, we must recognize that shame can stem from various experiences and aspects of our lives. For many of my clients, their shame is rooted in childhood experiences, professional failures, or societal expectations they feel they've failed to meet.

As I continued to explore vulnerability in my personal life and professional practice, I began to see how closely intertwined it was with shame. To truly be vulnerable, we must be willing to face our shame head-on. This is no easy task, as shame often feels like a heavy, suffocating blanket that we'd rather keep hidden away.

It's also important to understand the difference between shame and guilt as they are often confused. Feelings of guilt translate into "I did something wrong" (for example, cheating on one's partner). The experience of shame is quite different. We experience shame internally: "I am a bad person—there is something wrong with me."

Recognizing this distinction is crucial in your journey towards vulnerability. Guilt can often be a catalyst for positive change, prompting you to alter your behavior. Shame, on the other hand, can be paralyzing, causing you to retreat further into yourself and away from authentic connections.

One of my clients, Sarah, provided a powerful example of this distinction. Sarah had been struggling with intimacy issues in her relationship, always keeping her partner at arm's length. During our sessions, she revealed that she had been sexually abused as a child by a family member. For years, she had carried the weight of this experience, believing that she was somehow to blame, that there was something inherently wrong with her.

"I've always felt so dirty," she confessed, tears welling up in her eyes, "like I'm damaged goods. How could anyone truly love me if they knew?"

This was classic shame talk. Sarah wasn't feeling guilty about something she had done; she was feeling shame about who she believed she was at her core.

Over the course of our work together, we focused on helping Sarah understand that the abuse wasn't her fault. We worked on separating her sense of self from the traumatic experience she had endured as a child. We also worked on helping her learn how to regulate her nervous system so she could notice when she was feeling frozen; and I also provided her with numerous tools to help her regain her sense of safety in her body.

## Shame Thrives through Secrecy, Silence, and Judgment

In her book, Brown identifies three elements that allow shame to thrive: secrecy, silence, and judgment. In Sarah's case, the sexual abuse she experienced as a child, although revealed to her parents, was otherwise kept secret since it would have impacted family relations. Unfortunately, this is a very common experience, especially when the abuser is a member of the family. As a result, she was barely able to share this information with her partner and did not disclose the full extent of the abuse to anyone until she started working with me. The judgment that Sarah felt was internal, and it caused her to experience low self-esteem, misplaced self-guilt, and feeling unworthy of being loved. Sarah also held the not uncommon, yet false belief that she would be negatively judged by others if she disclosed her childhood abuse. This kind of belief also perpetuates the secrecy and silence, creating a shame spiral.

## Vulnerability Is the Antidote to Shame

While shame can block you from being vulnerable with your partner, the paradox is that it is only through vulnerability that we can banish or at least diminish our shame. Let's explore the three elements necessary to banish shame and embrace vulnerability:

- Recognizing a Shame Response
- Normalizing the Experience
- Self-Compassion and Empathy

## How does Shame Show Up in Your Body?

It's often challenging to recognize that you're feeling shame. Shame has a way of creeping up on us, often when we're not even expecting it. A lot of individuals experience shame during sex due to body image or performance issues. It causes them to shut down, but they're not really aware in the moment that what they are experiencing is shame. The more adept you become at recognizing a shame response occurring in your body, the faster you will be able to meet it and use your vulnerability skills to banish or diminish it.

## *Somatic Shame Exercise*

1. Find a quiet place where you can be undisturbed for a few minutes.
2. Close your eyes, take a few deep breaths, and feel your feet on the floor.
3. Identify a memory or experience that you feel some shame about. It does not have to be sexual. Please avoid using a significantly traumatic memory or experience.
4. Allow yourself to really be in that memory, creating it as vividly as you can in your mind. Notice where you are, what your age is, who else is in this memory, and exactly what happened. Play the memory out in slow motion as if it's a video on your phone.
5. Now begin to notice what's happening in your body as you replay this memory. What sensations are you noticing (heat, warmth, dizziness, tightness, cold, chills, shaking, stomachache, and so on), and where in your body are these sensations showing up? Stay in this memory only long enough for you to take note of your physical (or somatic) experience.
6. Open your eyes, shake your hands and move your body, and write down what you experienced in your body with as much specificity as possible.

Was this a familiar feeling in your body? At what other times have you experienced it? This is how your body reacts to shame.

In my own life, I've experienced a lot of sexual shame; I can now recognize that quickly in my body and banish it. However, I've recently come to realize the extent to which I have internalized shame due to the constant criticism by my mother when I was growing up. This showed up for me during a tense moment with my partner Daren when I was feeling heavily criticized by him and judged for a decision I made. At that moment, I felt a wave of heat wash over my body; I dissociated and wanted to crawl under the carpet.

I took a few breaths, looked straight at him, and disclosed, "I'm feeling a lot of shame right now by the way you're talking to me. It's triggering my wounds from being criticized by my mother so much." To his credit, he didn't get defensive (one of his frequent coping strategies). Instead, he took me in his arms, held me while I cried, and gently said, "I can see how much that hurts you. I accept you, Xanet, exactly how you are, and I love all parts of you". With those words of empathy, my nervous system was re-regulated, and we were able to calmly repair our conflict.

### Normalizing Your Shame

Since silence and secrecy are the ingredients that perpetuate the shame cycle, to banish shame, we need to normalize our lived experience for which we were shamed. This is where vulnerability becomes so critical. You can't normalize your experience of shame without being able to share it with someone else. Sharing about what occurred with my dog Lucky was the process by which my experience of shame became normalized. In fact, when I shared this story with a large group in a women's retreat, several women came up to me afterwards and told me they'd had similar experiences with their dogs and cats growing up. A huge sense of relief washed over me as I understood, for the first time, that I was not weird or broken and that this was a fairly normal experience for young girls.

## SELF-COMPASSION AND EMPATHY

Finding compassion for yourself can be very challenging. I always like to remind myself and my clients that we're human, and we make mistakes. None of us can escape from that essential truth. Also, many of our shame experiences happen *to* us and are outside of our control, such as going through sexual abuse, or getting an erection in public, which many teenage boys involuntarily experience.

Cultivating compassion and self-acceptance is a crucial step in overcoming shame and embracing vulnerability. For many of my clients, this is one of the most challenging aspects of their journey. They've spent years, sometimes decades, berating themselves for perceived flaws or past mistakes. Learning to treat themselves with kindness and understanding often feels foreign and uncomfortable at first.

**Body Shame Case Study: Jordan and Sarah**

One of my clients, Jordan, was struggling with intimacy issues in his marriage. In one of our sessions, he revealed his deep-seated shame about his body, especially the size of his penis. This was impacting his ability to have an erection, and he was even considering a penile implant. When I gently questioned Jordan about the source of his distress, he said that he had overheard his wife Sarah and a girlfriend talking about how much they loved big cocks. Jordan also spent a fair amount of time watching porn and was comparing himself to the male porn stars, whose penis sizes are typically in the 90 percent range.

I had Jordan measure his erect penis, which fell squarely in the normal range of 6 inches. (The length of the average erect penis is 5.16 inches.) While this information helped Jordan normalize his penis size, we also had to work on his self-compassion and acceptance that his penis was perfect just the way it was.

At our next couples session, I asked Jordan to vulnerably share with his partner some shame he was experiencing during sex.

Jordan hesitated, his eyes darting nervously around the room. I could see the internal struggle playing out on his face—the desire to be honest warring with his fear of being judged. Finally, he took a deep breath and turned to face his wife, Sarah.

"I...I've been feeling really ashamed about my body," he began, his voice barely above a whisper. "Especially...especially about the size of my penis."

Sarah's eyes widened in surprise, but she remained silent, allowing Jordan to continue.

"I overheard you talking with your friend about how much you love big...well, you know," he said, his cheeks flushing. "And I've been watching porn and comparing myself to those guys. I know it's not realistic, but I can't help feeling inadequate."

Jordan's voice cracked slightly as he finished, "I've been so worried that I'm not enough for you and that I've been disappointing you for all these years."

Sarah reached out and took Jordan's hand.

"Oh, honey," she said gently. "I had no idea you heard that conversation. I'm so sorry it hurt you."

Sarah's eyes welled with tears as she continued, "I want you to know that I love your body, all of it. The size of your penis has never been an issue for me. What matters to me is the connection we share, the intimacy we have."

She paused, taking a deep breath before adding, "I'm ashamed, too, now that we're talking about it. I could imagine that might feel disrespectful to you and our relationship."

Jordan looked up, meeting Sarah's gaze for the first time since he started speaking. The acceptance and love he saw there made his chest tighten with emotion.

"I had no idea you were carrying this burden," Sarah said softly. "Thank you for being brave enough to share it with me. I love you, Jordan. All of you."

As I watched this exchange, I could see the tension visibly leaving Jordan's face and tears of relief falling down his cheeks.

## *Facing Shame: A Partner Exercise*

This exercise provides you and your partner an opportunity to slowly reveal embarrassing and shameful moments in your life without judgment. The key element is to go slow—-revealing shame is like peeling an onion, exposing one layer at a time.

1. Find a quiet space where you can be undisturbed for ten minutes. Take a few minutes to write down on a piece of paper some things that you are ashamed or embarrassed about.
2. The first person faces their partner and reveals something that is embarrassing for them.
Example: "I'm feeling ashamed about how much weight I've gained and how much I hate what my body looks like."
3. The second partner listens and responds with empathy.
"I'm sorry you're feeling bad about your body. I know how hard it is to feel that way. I've felt that way too at times."

*Note:* It's critically important not to try to fix this (which can sound like, "Why don't you try that new exercise program I told you about?") or invalidate your partner's feelings by disagreeing with them (even if it is a compliment like, "I think your body is perfect"). Remember empathy means that you're standing in your partner's shoes for the moment. You are not judging them; you are only recognizing their pain and shame, and if appropriate, helping to normalize it by relating it to your own experience.

4. Switch roles, and then continue to go back and forth so that each person has at least five opportunities to express some embarrassment and shame.
5. Discuss what this experience was like for each of you. Notice if

anything shifts for you as you continue to normalize your shame experience.

## CULTIVATING VULNERABILITY IN YOUR RELATIONSHIP

### DO YOUR OWN WORK

Vulnerability requires a level of self-awareness around your own fears and wounds. As I can attest, this is easier said than done and may require obtaining some help through counseling, coaching, or self-development workshops. I also highly recommend journaling as a way to explore your own emotional patterns and challenges.

I'm personally a fan of the Morning Pages journaling process used in *The Artist's Way* by Julia Cameron. The goal is to write three pages a day, first thing upon waking. This is extemporaneous writing, recording your stream-of-consciousness thoughts. Think of it as a brain dump to clear your mind and allow more conscious emotions to arise.

You can write about anything that comes to mind, but this is not your to-do list. Importantly, you do not go back, at least not initially, to read this, and there is no editing. Also, do not use a computer—-there is a flow to writing by hand, even if your handwriting is incomprehensible. According to Cameron, writing the three pages helps to push past surface level chatter and delve deeper into thoughts and emotions.

### CREATE A SAFE ENVIRONMENT

To cultivate vulnerability in your relationship, it's important to ensure that both you and your partner are fully on board and adopt this as a shared value. Naturally, as two humans, you will inevitably push each other's buttons; and moments of vulnerability may be quickly discarded when your inner child takes control.

This is normal and is to be expected until you both master the skills to slow everything down and learn how to reconnect. When this occurs, I recommend that you go back to Chapter 3 and practice some of the exercises around connection. I often find that when Daren and I need to slow down and reconnect, spending five minutes of eye gazing, without words, can help settle both of our nervous systems and allow us to move into a more vulnerable space.

## Improve Your Emotional IQ

Vulnerability can't be fostered until you and your partner can authentically and honestly share feelings. One of the roadblocks to expressing your feelings is not having a lexicon of "feeling words." I find that most of my clients get really stuck when I ask them what they are feeling and often revert to something like "I'm feeling bad."

Let's go back to Jordan and Sarah as they start to navigate how to create more vulnerability in their relationship. When they arrived in my office, I could tell from the looks on their faces that trouble was brewing.

I invited Jordan and Sarah to sit down, noting the tension between them. "What's been going on since our last session?" I asked gently.

Sarah spoke first, her voice tight with frustration. "We've been trying to be more open with each other, like you suggested. But it feels like we're just going in circles. Jordan keeps saying he's 'fine' when I know something's bothering him."

Jordan sighed, running a hand through his hair. "I'm trying, I really am. But every time I start to open up, I freeze. I don't know how to put what I'm feeling into words."

I nodded, understanding their struggle. "This is actually quite common. Many people struggle to identify and express their emotions accurately. Let's try an exercise to expand your emotional vocabulary. I'd like to introduce you to one of my favorite tools; it's called an Emotions Wheel, and it will help you identify what emotion you're experiencing and how it relates to one of the four core human emotions: mad, sad, glad, and scared."

I pulled out a colorful circular diagram and placed it on the coffee table between us. Sarah and Jordan leaned forward, their curiosity piqued.

"This wheel breaks down emotions into more specific feelings," I explained. "For example, 'mad' can be further broken down into frustrated, irritated, or resentful. 'Sad' might be disappointed, lonely, or discouraged. The second layer of the wheel identifies the secondary emotions related to the core emotions, and the third layer of the wheel identifies the tertiary layer of emotions."

Jordan studied the wheel intently. "Huh. I never realized there were so many different ways to describe how I'm feeling."

Sarah nodded, her finger tracing the various sections. "This is fascinating. I can see how some emotions I thought were separate are actually related."

"Exactly," I said. "Now, I'd like each of you to think about how you're feeling right now, at this moment. Use the wheel to help you pinpoint the emotion."

Sarah took a deep breath and looked at the wheel. "I think I'm feeling...frustrated. But also, underneath that, maybe a bit anxious?"

I nodded encouragingly. "Good, Sarah. Can you elaborate on why you're feeling those emotions?"

She paused, considering. "I'm frustrated because I want us to connect more deeply, but it feels like we're stuck. And I guess I'm anxious because...well, what if we can't get past this?"

I turned to Jordan. "What about you, Jordan? What emotions are you experiencing right now?"

Jordan studied the wheel intently, his brow furrowed in concentration. After a moment, he spoke softly. "I think I'm feeling... overwhelmed. And maybe a little ashamed."

"That's great insight, Jordan," I said. "Can you tell us more about those feelings?"

He nodded slowly. "I'm feeling so much pressure from Sarah to share my feelings and try to be vulnerable. It's so uncomfortable for me that I just want to avoid talking to her so I don't have to deal with this. I'm also ashamed that I can't do it well."

"That's totally understandable, Jordan," I said. "Vulnerability can be really challenging; it's a new muscle for you that hasn't been flexed. But just sharing how you're feeling about this with Sarah is a big step towards more vulnerability."

Sarah reached out and gently touched Jordan's arm. "I had no idea you were feeling so overwhelmed," she softly said. "I'm sorry if I've been putting too much pressure on you."

Jordan looked at her, surprise evident in his eyes. "You're not mad?"

Sarah shook her head. "No, I'm not mad. I'm actually feeling...grateful that you shared that with me. And maybe a little guilty that I didn't realize how hard this has been for you."

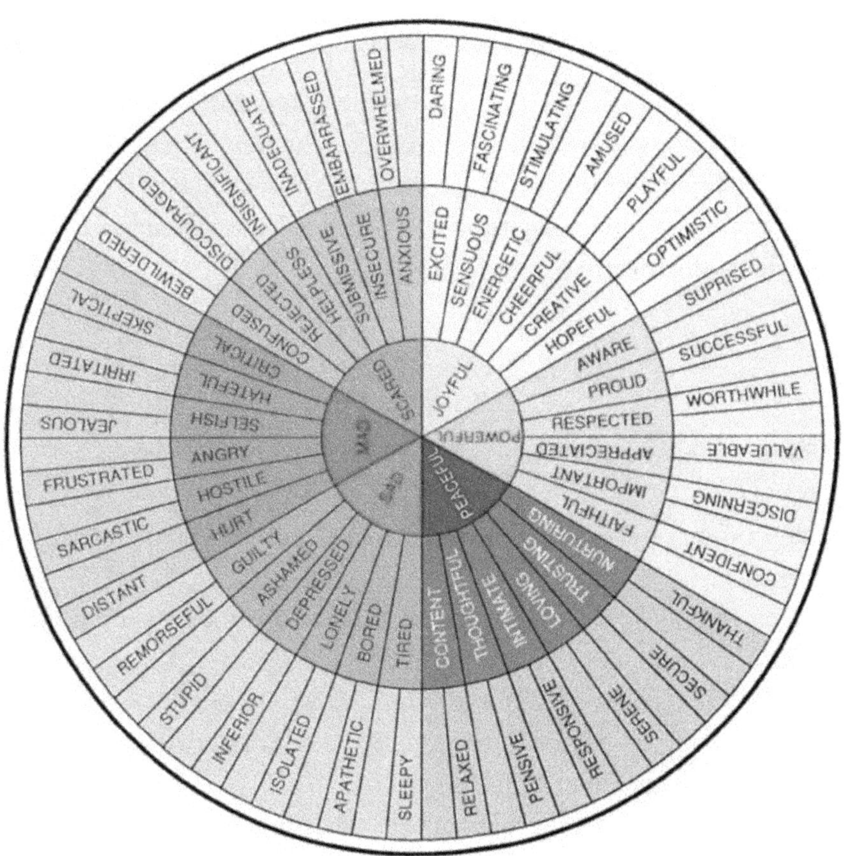


The Feeling Wheel

I SMILED, WATCHING THE INTERACTION BETWEEN THEM. "THIS IS EXACTLY the kind of open communication we're aiming for. Jordan, you were able to identify and express your feelings, and Sarah, you responded with empathy and understanding."

"Now," I continued, "let's practice using this emotions wheel regularly. Each day, try to check in with each other and share how you're feeling using the more specific terms from the wheel. Remember that this practice is about listening to your partner with empathy and validating their feelings."

## *Feeling Wheel Exercise*

1. Find a quiet space where you will not be interrupted for ten minutes.
2. Close your eyes, take a few deep breaths, and feel your feet on the ground.
3. Open your eyes, face your partner, and establish some eye contact.
4. The first person looks at the emotions wheel and tells their partner what feelings they are having and the context around the feeling (perhaps using an "I" statement like, "I'm feeling frustrated that you didn't help me clean up after dinner").
5. The second person reflects back what they heard their partner say with empathy (example: "Sounds like you're really frustrated with me that I didn't help clean the dishes. I can totally understand your frustration. Thanks for sharing your feelings").

The only job here is to validate your partner's feelings—not to judge, become defensive, or try to fix things.

6. Switch roles.
7. After you've both had a chance to share, you can explore whether there were any overlaps or patterns (example: "I can see that we're both feeling unappreciated by each other").

I recommend that couples do this exercise several times a week to build their communication and vulnerability skills.

**Vulnerability Enhances Your Sex Life**

The third and final section of this book delves into the realm of deepening sexual intimacy with your partner, offering a wealth of tools and techniques to enhance your connection and cultivate a lifelong bond of passionate intimacy. It is important to note that vulnerability is the foundation upon which true sexual satisfaction, exploration, and playful experimentation are built. It requires trust and openness, allowing yourself to be fully known and accepted by your partner. Together, you will discover new levels of pleasure, connection, and erotic discovery that will last a lifetime.

# 7
# BUILDING EMOTIONAL RESILIENCE THROUGH RELATIONSHIP REPAIR

Whenever I have the chance to meet couples in truly happy relationships, ones that have stood the test of time, I never fail to ask them what their secret is. Without fail, the answer that comes up most often is their ability to face challenges head-on and emerge stronger from conflict and hardship. These couples have built a deep well of emotional resilience that nourishes and sustains their bond, keeping it healthy and vibrant through the years.

The manner in which couples create emotional resilience can vary. Sometimes it occurs when they are forced to deal with health challenges, troubling family dynamics, or catastrophic events. These types of events can either bring couples together as they prioritize the need to work as a team, or they can tear a couple apart. The pandemic was the perfect petri dish. The experience of being quarantined with one's partner for months at a time helped strengthen the bonds of resilient couples but significantly weakened or ruptured the bonds of those with less stability in their relationships.

Creating and maintaining emotional resilience is a foundational element for sustaining intimacy in a long-term relationship.

Emotional resilience creates safety and trust since there is a shared belief that no matter what challenges arise, you will face them together and come out stronger.

**Case Study: Amy and Glenn** Meet Amy and Glenn. They have been married for thirty-five years, and when they were about to reach semi-retirement, Amy was diagnosed with a very rare genetic disease. For months, they struggled to find answers about her deteriorating health and had to cope with the unknown as they watched Amy go from being a robust and lively woman to someone who struggled to climb a flight of stairs without getting out of breath. While this could have driven a wedge between them, it actually created more connection and intimacy in their relationship. Glenn not only became Amy's advocate in navigating the health care system, but through his internet research and relentless pursuit of answers, he eventually found a specialist who was able to diagnose and treat Amy's condition. Throughout this ordeal, they learned to communicate more openly about their fears and vulnerabilities, deepening their emotional connection.

As Amy's health improved, they reflected on how this challenge had transformed their relationship. "It was like we rediscovered each other," Amy shared. "Seeing Glenn fight so hard for me, it made me fall in love with him all over again."

Glenn nodded in agreement. "We've always been close, but this experience taught us how to truly lean on each other. It's not just about the good times anymore; it's about facing the tough times together and coming out stronger."

## Filling Up Your Appreciation Bucket

A fairly easy way to build emotional resilience and to help your partner to feel seen and heard is through making the time for appreciations. It's not uncommon in long-term relationships to at some point begin to take your partner for granted, expecting that they will always be there doing the things they've always done. But actively expressing appreciation for your partner, even for the small things, can have a profound impact on your relationship.

Not only do appreciations make your partner feel validated and valued, but they also help to temper any criticisms that might arise in the relationship, a not uncommon occurrence. I have a rule of thumb that for every one criticism, you must give your partner five appreciations. It is important to recognize that filling up each other's appreciation bucket is an important step towards creating more emotional resilience.

Amy and Glenn incorporated this practice into their daily check-in routine during Amy's health scare. Every evening, they would share at least one thing they appreciated about each other from that day. Sometimes it was as simple as Glenn thanking Amy for making his favorite breakfast, or Amy expressing gratitude for Glenn remembering to pick up her prescription.

"It's amazing how such a small gesture can make such a big difference," Amy reflected. "There were days during my illness when I felt utterly useless, but hearing Glenn's appreciations reminded me that I still had value, that I was still contributing to our partnership."

Glenn added, "And for me, it helped me notice all the little things Amy does that I might have overlooked before. It made me more mindful of how much she contributes to my life and our marriage."

## *Appreciation Exercise*

1. Find a quiet space without any interruptions.
2. Face your partner, close your eyes, and take a few breaths.
3. Open your eyes and establish eye contact.
4. The person who is going first gives their partner five to seven

appreciations. I recommend that these are items that are not just surface but rather ones that come from the heart. Also, the more details you provide, the more likely the appreciation will register. There's a big difference between telling your partner, "I appreciate your body," as opposed to "I love touching your shoulders because they feel so solid and strong, just like you."

5. The person receiving the appreciations really takes it in and notices where they feel it in their body. Be sure to acknowledge your partner for all of their appreciations.
6. Switch roles with your partner.
7. Take a few moments to discuss and process any feelings that arise.

Additional ways to fill up your appreciation jar:

- Add an appreciation to your daily check-in.
- Create an "appreciation jar" where you drop in written appreciations daily, using different colored paper for each of you.

## RELATIONSHIP RUPTURES ARE NORMAL

Every so often I'll meet a couple who tells me, "We never have an argument or fight." When I hear that, I know this is likely not a healthy relationship and that underneath their surface congeniality, there is deep resentment, anger, and years of unprocessed disappointment and hurt. The reality is that conflict is normal and healthy in an intimate relationship. There is no possible way that two individuals with different personalities and life experiences are always going to agree with each other's opinions and be able to meet all of each other's desires and needs. The key is not to avoid conflict, but to learn how to navigate it in a way that strengthens the relationship and enhances connection and intimacy.

As we discussed in Chapter 2, ruptures in relationships can occur for a variety of reasons, including miscommunication, not feeling seen or heard, feeling judged by your partner, unresolved conflicts and resentments, and life stressors, to name just a few.

Many conflicts are seemingly small, such as getting annoyed at your partner for not taking the trash out. This is similar to a little scratch on your finger that doesn't even need a Band-Aid. But underlying that emotional 'scratch' is a feeling of disappointment and maybe even a bit of disrespect. Over time, these small ruptures begin to grow, and that little scratch starts to fester until eventually it becomes a nasty wound.

Other conflicts can be more significant and cut more deeply. These might include disagreements about major life decisions, financial issues, or differing values and goals. Then of course there are the major relationship traumas—infidelity and betrayal—that will require significant rehabilitation if the relationship is to survive.

**Case Study: Mia and Rosalyn**

Take the case of Mia and Rosalyn, who have been together for a decade. On the surface, their relationship appeared perfect. They rarely argued and always presented a united front to the world. However, beneath this facade of harmony, a storm was brewing.

Mia had been harboring frustration for years over Rosalyn's tendency to prioritize work over their relationship. She'd mention it casually, but Rosalyn would brush it off, assuming it wasn't a big deal since Mia never raised her voice or initiated a serious discussion about it.

One day, the dam finally broke. Rosalyn came home late; having completely forgotten she had promised to take Mia out to celebrate her winning an award for her artwork. When Rosalyn arrived home, two hours late, she was met with a note on the door that said Mia was staying with her sister until further notice and Rosalyn was not to contact her.

A week later, they landed in my office, in significant distress and on the verge of separation. As I sat across from Mia and Rosalyn for the very first time, the tension between them was palpable. Mia's arms were crossed tightly over her chest, her eyes red-rimmed from crying. Rosalyn sat on the other side of the couch, looking bewildered and defeated.

"I just don't understand," Rosalyn began, her voice tinged with frustration. "We've always gotten along so well. Why didn't you tell me how upset you were?"

Mia's laugh was bitter. "I've been telling you for years, Rosalyn. You just never listened."

As we delved deeper into their history, it became clear that their picture-perfect relationship had been built on a foundation of avoidance and unspoken resentments. Mia had learned to swallow her disappointment, believing that a "good" relationship meant never fighting. Rosalyn, accustomed to this dynamic, had grown complacent, mistaking silence for contentment.

Over the next few sessions, we started to unpack some of the resentments that had been built up over the last decade. The list was long but continued to repeat the same pattern, as is common in all relationships. Rosalyn felt ignored by Mia and didn't feel loved or desired, and Mia felt that Rosalyn never put her on the top of her priority list, choosing to spend her time working and hanging out with her friends from work on the weekend.

As we worked through these issues, I encouraged Mia and Rosalyn to practice expressing their needs and frustrations in real time using the emotions wheel, rather than bottling them up. It was a challenging process, filled with heated discussions and moments of vulnerability that left them both feeling raw and exposed.

One particularly intense session stands out in my memory. Rosalyn, finally grasping the depth of Mia's hurt, broke down in tears. "I never meant to make you feel unimportant," she said, her voice choked with emotion. "I thought I was providing for us, building a future. But I see now that I was building it alone, not with you."

Mia, moved by Rosalyn's vulnerability, reached out and took her hand. It was the first physical contact I'd seen between them. "And I should have been clearer about how I was feeling," she admitted. "I was so afraid of rocking the boat that I just continued to swallow all of my disappointments and tell myself that's just what marriage is like. My parent's marriage was similar...Dad worked all the time, and Mom just put up with it. My father never had time for me either."

"Mia," I said gently, "you just revealed an important piece of information."

"What do you mean?" Mia asked, her brow furrowed in confusion.

I leaned forward slightly, my voice soft but firm. "You mentioned your parents' relationship and how your father was often absent. It's likely that this experience from your childhood has influenced your expectations and fears in your own marriage."

Rosalyn turned to Mia, her eyes widening with realization. "Is that why you never pushed harder when I was working late? Were you afraid I'd leave if you confronted me?"

Mia's eyes welled up with tears. "I...I guess I was. I always told myself that's just how things were, that I should be grateful for what I had. But deep down, I was terrified of you abandoning me, just like my father had emotionally abandoned me."

This revelation marked a turning point in our work. Over the next few sessions, we explored how both Mia and Rosalyn's perception of what intimacy should look like was based on how their parents had modeled it for each of them. We also identified how in some ways they had each chosen a partner who mirrored aspects of their parents' relationships, unconsciously recreating familiar patterns.

This is a very common experience for couples. We tend to choose partners who demonstrate love in ways similar to how our parents demonstrated love, even if it was unhealthy. We also tend to choose partners who have similar emotional patterns to our parents and who trigger our deepest childhood wounds, because this feels familiar and comfortable, even if it's dysfunctional. However, rather than this being the death knell to a relationship, it actually provides the opportunity for healing and growth as you begin to understand how to break the pattern by changing your behaviors and communicating in a more effective manner.

## RELATIONSHIP REPAIR SKILLS

If you're like most couples, it's likely that when you and your partner get into an altercation, one of you attempts to repair it in the heat of the argument. Not only is this completely ineffective, but it generally results in escalation of the conflict. I'm about to share with you the secret to creating and maintaining a healthy relationship, so please pay close attention to this section.

Drum roll please...The secret to a healthy relationship is learning how to repair conflicts. That's it! If you can learn how to repair your relationship when conflicts arise, you're on the way to creating a healthy long-term relationship.

You might be asking yourself, "Xanet, why do we need to repair conflict? Isn't it fine if we both just apologize to each other and kiss and make up? It's been working for us so far." My response to that question: "Are you sure it's really working?" In reality, if you don't fully address the root of the conflict and instead only "patch up" the unresolved feelings, they will only continue to fester and grow over time. This can lead to resentment and discontent within the relationship. As a result, you feel emotionally disconnected from your partner, resulting in less desire for physical intimacy and sex. On the other hand, addressing and repairing conflict with your partner will create more emotional connection and safety as you both feel valued, seen, and heard.

If you've ever seen a couples therapist, you might be scratching your head and wondering why no one has ever taught you how to repair conflicts. It's the same question that I continue to ask myself every single time that I'm working with a couple on one of my retreats and they tell me, "We have been to see many couple therapists, and we have never heard about a repair process." Perhaps this process is rarely included in master's degree counseling and therapy programs. Or maybe this is just a fundamental difference between the therapy and coaching models. As a sex and intimacy coach, my goal is to diagnose the issue, provide clients with skills, help them reach their achievable goals, and then set them free. The therapy model seems to be more focused on therapy sessions being the mechanism for conflict resolution.

Luckily for you, Danielle Harel and Celeste Hirschman, the cofounders of the Somatica Institute, have created an excellent relationship repair process that I teach to all my clients. This section of the book will draw broadly from the Somatica Relationship Repair Process. A link to the complete article on the Somatica Process, "9 Steps to Relationship Repair", is found in the References section at the end of the book.

## Acknowledging Your Shortcomings

Mia and Rosalyn were making good progress on communicating more openly with each other, so I decided it was time to teach them some of the steps involved in relationship repair.

After they were settled in my office, this time actually sitting next to each other on my couch, I turned to them and said, "I want to tell you a story about the first time Daren and I met." They looked up with quizzical looks on their faces. "At the end of my first date with Daren, I told him, I want you to know all of the ways in which it can be extra frustrating to be in a relationship with me. He was surprised but listened attentively. I then proceeded to list the following reasons:

- I can be judgmental
- I can be controlling
- I can be demanding
- I can be impatient
- I can be very anxiously attached
- I can be selfish
- I have an abandonment wound

"Wow," Mia exclaimed, "what did he say after that?"

"He thanked me for sharing and told me he appreciates a woman who really understands herself. In truth, this is just a partial list, but I didn't want to totally scare him away," I said with a chuckle. "Then I asked him the same question, and he revealed a few things about his relationship with his father, but it wasn't until about a year later that I got the full picture," I said with a raised eyebrow. Mia and Rosalyn laughed and visibly relaxed.

"Now I want each of you to write down on a piece of paper all of the ways in which it's challenging to be in a romantic relationship with you."

Mia and Rosalyn looked at each other nervously before picking up their pens. For several minutes, the only sound in the room was the scratching of pen on paper. I watched as their expressions shifted from concentration to moments of wry amusement and even flashes of shame.

“All right,” I said after they both set down their pens. “Now, I'd like you to share what you've written with each other.”

Rosalyn cleared her throat and began. “Well, I can be stubborn and set in my ways. I have a hard time admitting when I'm wrong. I tend to shut down emotionally when things get tough instead of talking about my feelings. I can be a workaholic and often prioritize my job over our relationship. And...I'm not always the best listener.”

Mia nodded, a mix of emotions playing across her face. Her voice trembled slightly as she began to read from her list. “I can be passive-aggressive instead of directly expressing my needs. I tend to bottle up my emotions until I explode. I have a hard time trusting that people won't leave me, so I sometimes push them away first. I can be overly critical and a perfectionist. And...I struggle with vulnerability and often hide behind a facade of being ‘fine’ when I'm not.”

As Mia finished reading, she looked up at Rosalyn, her eyes glistening with unshed tears. Rosalyn reached out and took her hand, squeezing it gently.

I let the moment settle before speaking. “Thank you both for your honesty. This exercise is crucial because it helps you recognize your own contributions to relationship challenges. It's easy to focus on our partner's faults, but true growth comes from acknowledging your own.”

Mia looked at Rosalyn and said gently, “It felt really validating to hear you acknowledge some of your behaviors. It made me feel like I’m not crazy because it seems like you can never admit that you’re wrong about anything.”

Rosalyn nodded, a look of understanding crossing her face. "I can see how frustrating that must be for you. I guess I've always had a hard time admitting my faults because I was afraid it would make me seem weak or incompetent. But hearing you share your own challenges...it makes me realize we're both just human, trying our best."

"Exactly," I interjected. "And that's a key part of building emotional resilience in your relationship. By acknowledging your own shortcomings, you create a space where both of you can be vulnerable and authentic. Hold onto this paper," I said, "We're going to be using it at our next session when I teach you the repair process."

## *Self-Awareness of Your Shortcomings Exercise:*

1. Find a quiet space and make sure you have paper and pen.
2. Spend a few minutes writing about what makes it challenging to be in a relationship with you. This can be a list of your personality traits ("I can be intense"), behaviors ("I can be controlling"), baggage ("I have a hard time trusting others"), and/or wounds ("I can be avoidant"). Be kind and compassionate to yourself, because you are an imperfect human being just like the rest of us, but also be as honest as possible. If you can connect any of your behaviors to your childhood wounds, write that down as well. You might want to go back and refer to Chapter 3.
3. Read your lists aloud to your partner, making sure that you remain an active listener when your partner is speaking, but without interrupting or editorializing.
4. Discuss and process the experience with your partner.

Think about the emotions that surfaced when your partner opened up about their own struggles.

# THE REPAIR PROCESS

**Step 1: Identify the Emotional Conversation Under the Conflict.**

One of the reasons that couples struggle to resolve conflicts is that they mistakenly believe that they are arguing about the facts. This places them in an adversarial situation where they try unsuccessfully to debate each other, each believing their own version of the truth. In reality, there is an emotional conversation underlying the conflict, and without addressing those emotions, the conflict can never successfully be repaired.

To better explain my point, let me provide an example of the first big argument Daren and I had. I'd noticed that when Daren got in the car, he didn't buckle his seatbelt, and that unless I reminded him, he always seemed to "forget" to wear it. One day headed into downtown Asheville, I just had enough.

"It drives me crazy that you forget to put your seat belt on." Daren sighed, clearly frustrated. "I don't forget, I just don't think it's necessary for short trips around town. You don't need to remind me every time we get in the car."

I felt my anger rising. "It's the law! And it's not safe. Do you not care about your own safety? We live on a narrow, curvy, two-lane road with construction trucks flying down the mountain. And bears and deer come out of nowhere! What if you must slam on the brakes?"

"I've worked in the ER and ICU for decades," he exclaimed, "and I'm certain that if I'm driving under 35 mph, no one's going to get killed. And if we're hit by a truck head-on, we're goners anyway, regardless of whether we're wearing seat belts."

We went back and forth like this for several minutes, each of us reciting our "facts" to support our position as our nervous systems became increasingly activated. When we got home, I took a walk around the neighborhood to calm myself down while he retreated to his peaceful sanctuary: the hot tub.

During my walk I asked myself, “What’s really going on here? What are the feelings that I’m having, and why am I so triggered?” Once I was clear on my own feelings and had calmed down from my trigger going off, I returned to the house, and Daren and I calmly sat down to talk.

“I realize now that when I nag you about not wearing your seatbelt, it’s not really about the seatbelt at all. I’m terrified that you’re going to get hurt and I’m going to lose you, just like I lost my father. I want to do everything in my power to prevent that from happening again.”

Daren's expression softened as he listened to my words. He reached out and took my hand, his eyes filled with understanding. “I had no idea that's what was behind your concern,” he said softly. “I know how deeply your father’s death affected you, and I can see now how my not wearing my seatbelt triggered all your fears of being abandoned.”

He paused for a moment, gathering his thoughts. “You know, I think I react so strongly to being told what to do because it reminds me of my father. He was always so controlling, always telling me how to live my life. When you remind me about the seatbelt, part of me feels like that little boy again, rebelling against authority.”

I squeezed his hand, feeling a wave of empathy wash over me. “I never meant to make you feel that way. I guess we both have some old wounds that are still affecting us.”

We sat in silence for a moment, letting the weight of our realizations settle between us.

He wrapped his arms around me, and we held each other tightly, taking long, deep breaths. Once again, I felt a sense of reconnection and safety with him.

This scenario demonstrates what I tell all my clients about conflicts. The facts are irrelevant. You can argue about them endlessly, but not only will you never feel satisfied, it will make you feel more disconnected from your partner. Conflicts stem from emotions rather than facts. When you're in conflict with your partner, you're having an emotional conflict.

## Step 2: Assess Your Level of Activation

Now that you recognize that conflicts stem from emotions rather than facts, it makes sense that resolving a conflict will also involve having an emotional conversation with your partner. As you've been learning throughout this book, emotional conversations require a level of self-awareness and vulnerability that is inaccessible when either one of you is highly activated or triggered.

Since your emotional wounds stem from childhood, when that wound is triggered, it's like you are being transported back in time. Suddenly your adult self fades away and the wounded child within takes over. All the pain and hurt floods back in an overwhelming wave, and that inner child tries to protect itself by reverting to childhood behavior. This is why I tell my couples, "When you are triggered, there is no adult in the room." With no adult presence, repair is impossible.

On a physiological basis, when you feel threatened (either due to present reality or based on past trauma) the amygdala, the fear center in your brain, is activated, which causes the stress hormones cortisol and adrenaline to be released in the body. These hormones can cause a fight (anger or aggression), flight (avoidance or running away) or freeze (overwhelmed, numb, dissociative) reaction to occur. At the same time, the prefrontal cortex, which manages emotional regulation and logical thinking, shuts down, making it difficult to think clearly, solve any problems, or respond rationally.

No adult is in the room!

For most individuals, if your level of activation or trigger is higher than a three (on a scale of one to ten), you should not attempt to have a repair conversation. You must wait until both you and your partner are less activated.

While some individuals know when they are triggered, I find that many don't. It's therefore important for you to explore what happens in your body when you get triggered, because your body will react well before your brain does.

### *Activation Exercise:*

1. Choose a time when you are both feeling grounded and calm.
2. Ask your partner to say something to you that you know will be upsetting to you. Maybe it's the words you ask them to use or their tone of voice, but your request is for them to speak in some way by which you will feel triggered. Find a topic to work with that is not a major pain point in your relationship—something annoying but not *extremely* activating.
3. Notice what's happening in your body when you hear those words. What sensations are you having? Where do they show up? Some common ways in which the body reacts include feeling tightness in the chest or the belly, feeling warmth in the face, or feeling an arm or leg starting to fidget or bounce.
4. Identify what your level of activation is on a scale of one to ten. If the level is fairly low, ask your partner to make adjustments until you can feel an increase in activation.

5. Switch which of you is doing the talking.
6. Discuss and share what you learned.

It's also important for you to understand what needs to happen for your nervous system to settle down. This can vary widely, and it's important not to question or judge what you or your partner needs. Also, the higher level of the activation, the more time and space you might need to de-escalate. Some common de-escalation tools include taking a walk, exercising, talking to a friend, journaling, distractions (such as video games or scrolling the web on a cell phone), and having alone time.

If you are more on the anxious attachment axis, you might be inclined to try to constantly check in with your partner while they are in the process of de-escalating. You might also try to immediately repair the conflict rather than feel the pain and fear of an attachment injury, since you are terrified that they will abandon you.

Engaging in either of these actions will probably only cause your partner to become more agitated, which is the opposite of what you are trying to achieve. This is why I always recommend that couples (1) tell their partner they are activated, (2) inform them of what they need to calm down, and (3) reassure their partner that they will let them know when they are ready to have a repair conversation.

## Step 3. Find the Right Time for the Repair Conversation

By nature of being an emotional conversation, repair conversations can take a bit of time, especially when you're just learning the process. I generally tell couples to allocate a minimum of thirty to forty-five minutes for these types of conversations. Therefore, it's critical that these conversations happen at the appropriate time.

Whoever decides that they are ready to repair should use words similar to these: "Are you open to having a repair conversation now?" This gives your partner an opportunity to both assess where they are both emotionally (for example, to evaluate, am I sufficiently recovered from my trigger?) and logistically (do I have time right now, or do I have to be at the office in half an hour or respond to some emails?). Again, it's important to wait until you are both totally prepared to have this conversation. If the time is not appropriate, it's incumbent on each partner to tell the other when they are available (for example, I'm free after seven, does that work for you too?).

Once you have truly created more vulnerability and emotional safety and resilience in your relationship, these repair conversations will be much more efficient. You will both be able to focus quickly on the essence of the emotional conversation and make repairs more quickly.

## Step 4. Remember That You're a Good Person

During a repair conversation, you are likely to hear your partner say some things that can make you feel uncomfortable or embarrassed or can even bring up some shame. So, before you get started, make sure that you remind yourself and your inner child that you are a good person, you are an imperfect human being as we all are, and you are doing the best you can.

## Step 5. Decide Who Goes First

Repair conversations are always two-sided, and it's not possible to have a productive conversation if both partner's emotions are aired at the same time. Also, while most repair conversations occur because a conflict has arisen that you are both aware of, there are times when this is not the case. For example, if your partner said or did something that upset you, but they are completely unaware of it, then you are the one who must start the repair conversation. In my own relationship, because I am a slow processor, it might take twenty-four hours for me to realize that something Daren said or did really triggered me. However, normally you can discuss who wants to go first. Sometimes it makes sense to allow the person who was more activated to start the repair, but this is completely your choice as a couple. If you notice that one person is always starting the repair conversation, you may need to examine that more closely, perhaps with the help of a coach or therapist.

## Step 6. Share Your Feelings Vulnerably

Here's the good news: If you've been practicing all the skills in this book so far, the next several steps will be familiar to you from Chapter 3. These are the key components of enhancing communication and building emotional intimacy.

The first person shares what they are feeling as a result of the conflict, using the emotions wheel if necessary. While you do need to provide your partner with a short summary of the facts, my rule of thumb is "less is more." It's easy to get caught up in the facts, but this will only serve to either trigger your partner more or make it really difficult for them to reflect back what they hear in the next step. Focus on the essence of your feelings; for example, "When you sprang on me the fact that your parents were coming to stay with us without checking in with me first, it made me feel insignificant, overwhelmed, and frustrated." It's important here to stay neutral and explain your feelings in a nonjudgmental, non-shaming way.

Pitfalls to Avoid:

- Do not judge, blame, or shame your partner. This is the reason you can't have an effective repair conversation when you're activated.
- To the very best of your ability, use "I" statements. There's a difference in saying "You made me feel sad" (blaming) versus "I felt sad."

## Step 7. Reflect Back with Empathy and Validate Your Partner's Feelings and Experience

The most challenging aspect of this step is being able to express empathy. While you worked on some empathy skills in Chapter 3, I want to offer you an opportunity to truly deepen your skills by engaging in one of my most impactful exercises, *Standing in Your Partner's Shoes.* This audio recording exercise, which can be accessed here https://www.passionateintimacyretreats.com/go-deeper/, is an opportunity to truly be seen and heard by your partner. I find this exercise an extremely useful practice for couples to experience empathy from their partner and build the necessary skills for Step 7 of the repair process:

While the first person shares their feelings vulnerably, the listener maintains eye contact and uses their active listening skills while being totally present with their partner. If the listener needs clarification, it's appropriate to ask a question once the first person has completed sharing vulnerably. What's not appropriate is to interrupt or correct your partner, especially around the facts, because doing so immediately invalidates them and will likely cause activation to occur.

Finding empathy for how your partner is feeling, regardless of your version of the facts, will make them feel heard and seen, which goes a long way towards repairing the conflict. Expressing empathy also helps prevent you from becoming defensive, which is a natural response when one feels attacked.

The listener should check in with their partner to ensure that their empathy landed. If it did not, then try again, or ask your partner what they need to hear. Be as specific as possible (for example, "the words were fine, but I didn't feel like you meant them").

During this step, it's important that the listener continues to track their own level of activation, which might rise, and informs their partner of what their new level might be. If it's risen too high, it might be wise to take a little break until they can calm down.

Pitfalls to Avoid:

- Do not editorialize and insert your own opinions, facts, or projections when reflecting back. Do your very best to really reflect back the essence of what your partner said and felt.
- With empathy, less is more. For example, "That must have really been terrible for you" might be just enough if said with compassion.
- Tone of voice is important. How you express empathy using your voice, body language, and eyes will be more important than the words you use.
- While it's fine to reference your own experience (example: "I know how painful it is to feel shame"), do not make this about you and start going into your own story. This immediately invalidates your partner's feelings.

## Step 8: Own Your Own Stuff

In this part of the repair process, the listener acknowledges their role in the conflict by owning up to one of their shortcomings that you identified in the Shortcoming Exercise. In the Somatica blog article, they call this "Cop to It." It's important, though, to distinguish between owning a behavior that makes it challenging to be in a relationship with you versus trying to apologize for what you did. Also, acknowledging your own behavior is never meant to be an excuse. It's an opportunity for you to acknowledge the impact of your behavioral pattern on your partner. It's also helpful to relate this pattern back to any childhood wounds that you've identified.

To go back to Daren and my conflict about the seatbelt, owning my own stuff would look like this: "I know that one of the challenges of being in a relationship with me is how intense my abandonment wound is and how I'm constantly trying to protect myself from that pain. I know it's really hard when I start to nag you because I'm trying to control you so that I don't have to feel the pain of possibly losing you. That's not fair to you, and I can see how it puts more pressure on you than necessary."

Pitfalls to Avoid:

- Watch out for your self-protective strategies. Focus on your partner's hurt, and do your best to continue to empathize with them. Breathe through any defensiveness that may come up. This is likely where your defenses will show up. The threat response is very real in this part of the conversation, so take a breath, and remember you're a good person doing your best.

## Step 9: Reassure Your Partner

In this step, the listener seeks to reassure their partner, once they truly understand what was upsetting them. It's important to only give a reassurance that is both truthful and something that you can live up to. Telling your partner "I'm sorry, I'll never do that again" is likely not a realistic promise because you are human, these patterns are ingrained, and you will likely repeat this. Unrealistic reassurances will only serve to further alienate your partner because they've probably heard that "promise" many times before. If the reassurance doesn't land, which is often the case, ask your partner what they would like to hear to reassure them. Then assess whether that's a reassurance you can honestly give them; if it is not, adjust the wording accordingly.

In the conversation with Daren, I would give him this reassurance. "I know how much you love me and that you have no intention of leaving me. I will continue to do my work in therapy, and the next time I get triggered, I'm going to take a few breaths and check in with myself before I react. I'll also try to communicate my fears more directly rather than nagging you about safety."

## Step 10: Switch Roles

Every conflict has two sides, and it's critically important that both of you have an opportunity to share your feelings. Also, it's not uncommon for something that was said during the first part of the repair conversation to trigger the listener, which then also must be repaired. The listener will follow the exact same steps identified above.

## Step 11: Evaluate

At the end of the repair process, discuss how you are both feeling. If the repair process was productive, there should be a feeling of some relief and hopefully a bit more emotional connection. But if one or both of you are still feeling activated, then it's likely that something got missed and some feelings are still unresolved. In that case, you may need to continue the repair process. Also, since we are often repairing unhealthy patterns in relationships, it's not at all uncommon that you will need to go back and repair the same conflict (or a similar variation of it—same feelings/different facts), several times.

**Repair Conversation: Mia and Rosalyn**

It's helpful to see how this actually plays out in real life. So, let's listen in on my session with Mia and Rosalyn where I took them through the repair process. I also want you to know that for educational purposes, I've crafted a straightforward repair conversation which never actually happens in a real session. In real life, we're constantly stopping and starting, especially as protective strategies keep showing up, so I want you to be realistic about what you can expect, especially the first several times that you try this.

"All right," I began, "let's start by identifying a recent conflict you two have had. Nothing too major for our first attempt, but something meaningful enough that it caused some tension between you."

Mia and Rosalyn exchanged glances before Mia spoke up. "Well, last weekend, Rosalyn promised to help me organize the garage. But when Saturday came, she spent most of the day working on a project for her job instead. I ended up doing most of the organizing by myself, and I was pretty upset about it."

Rosalyn nodded, a look of regret crossing her face. "Yeah, that's a good example. I know it really bothered you."

"Perfect conflict to address," I said. I also checked in to ensure that neither one of them were highly activated. "Mia, since you were most upset, why don't you start the repair?"

Mia turned toward Rosalyn and asked, "Rosalyn, are you open now to having a repair conversation about cleaning out the garage?" Rosalyn nodded her assent.

Mia took a deep breath and began. "When you didn't help me organize the garage like you promised, I felt really disappointed and unimportant. It brought up feelings of being neglected and not being a priority in your life." Her voice quivered slightly as she continued, "It reminded me of all the times my dad would cancel plans with me for work. I felt like I was that little girl again, always coming second to someone's job."

Rosalyn listened intently, her brow furrowed in concentration. When Mia finished, she paused for a moment before responding. "What I hear you saying is that when I chose to work instead of helping you with the garage, it made you feel neglected and unimportant. You felt like you weren't a priority to me, and it brought up painful memories of your dad always putting work before you. Is that right?"

Mia nodded. But I could tell something was still amiss. "That was a great reflection, Rosalyn, the only missing element was providing some empathy."

Rosalyn nodded, realizing her oversight. She took a deep breath and added, "I can imagine how painful that must have been for you, Mia—to feel like you were being pushed aside again, just like when you were a child. That must have felt really lonely and hurtful."

Mia's eyes welled up with tears. "Yes, that's exactly it. Thank you for understanding."

I nodded approvingly. "Great job, Rosalyn. Now, can you identify one of your shortcomings that contributed to this situation?"

Rosalyn thought for a moment. "Well, I guess this ties into what I wrote earlier about being a workaholic. I tend to prioritize work over other things, even when I've made commitments. It's a pattern I learned from my own father, always putting career first."

"That's good awareness, Rosalyn, but it also sounds a bit like an excuse," I gently added. Can you try saying that again, this time connecting it to its impact on Mia?"

She took a moment and then tried again. "Mia, one of the things that's challenging about being in a relationship with me is that I'm a workaholic. It must be really hard for you to feel like you're not a priority in my life, especially because your dad did the same thing to you."

"How did that land for you, Mia?" I gently asked. "That felt much better," she replied. "I have the sense that Rosalyn better understands now how her behavior impacts me."

"And how might you reassure Mia?" I prompted.

Rosalyn turned to Mia, taking her hand. "I want you to know that you are incredibly important to me. I realize now how my actions have been hurting you, and I'm committed to changing that. From now on, I will try to do a lot better when we make plans so that I can honor my commitment to our relationship. And if something urgent does come up, I'll do my best to communicate with you about it instead of just assuming you'll understand."

Mia squeezed her hand, a small smile forming on her lips. "Thank you, Rosalyn. That means a lot to me."

I nodded approvingly. "Excellent work, both of you. Now, Rosalyn, it's your turn to share your perspective on this conflict."

Rosalyn took a deep breath. "Mia, are you open to hearing my side of our conflict"? Mia nodded her head in agreement.

"When I didn't help with the garage like I promised, I felt really guilty and ashamed," Rosalyn began. "But underneath that, I was feeling overwhelmed and anxious about work. There's been a lot of pressure lately, and I worry that if I don't keep up, I might lose my job. That fear of failure...it's something that's always been with me."

I interrupted her for a moment. "Rosalyn, I'm curious about that last statement around your fear of failure. Do you have a sense of where that comes from?"

Rosalyn thought for a moment, “When I was growing up, I felt like my parents were always pushing me to do better and achieve more. Even though I was number two in my senior class, my parents were disappointed that I wasn’t the class valedictorian. So failing in anything, but especially my legal work, is not an option.”

Mia listened attentively, her expression softening as Rosalyn spoke. When she finished, Mia paused for a moment before responding. “What I hear you saying is that when you didn't help with the garage, you felt guilty and ashamed. But underneath that, you were feeling overwhelmed and anxious about work pressures. You have a deep fear of failure that comes from your parents’ high expectations. It wasn't that I'm not important to you, but that you were scared and falling into old patterns. Is that right?”

Rosalyn nodded, visibly relieved. “Yes, that's exactly it.”

Mia continued, her voice gentle, “I can imagine how stressful that must be for you, constantly feeling like you have to prove yourself through your work. It must be exhausting to carry that pressure all the time.”

“It really is,” Rosalyn admitted, her shoulders relaxing slightly.

I nodded approvingly. “Excellent, Mia. Now, can you identify one of your behaviors that contributed to this conflict?” Mia took a deep breath.

“One of the challenges of being in a relationship with me is that I tend to bottle up my emotions and not express my needs clearly,” Mia said, her voice soft but steady. “Instead of telling you directly how important it was to me that we work on the garage together, or how hurt I was feeling, I just got quiet and resentful. I realize now that this doesn't give you a fair chance to understand or meet my needs.”

Rosalyn listened intently, nodding in understanding. "Thank you for sharing that, Mia. It helps me understand your reaction better."

I smiled encouragingly at Mia. "That's great self-awareness, Mia. Now, how might you reassure Rosalyn?"

Mia turned to face Rosalyn fully, taking both her hands in hers. "Rosalyn, I want you to know that I understand the pressure you're under at work, and I don't want to add to that stress. I promise to communicate my needs and feelings more clearly in the future, instead of expecting you to read my mind. And I want you to know that I love you for who you are, not what you achieve."

Rosalyn's eyes glistened with emotion. "Thank you, Mia. That means so much to me."

I nodded approvingly. "Excellent work, both of you. Now, let's take a moment to evaluate how you're feeling after this repair process."

Mia spoke first. "I feel...lighter—like a weight has been lifted off my chest. I understand Rosalyn's perspective better now, and I feel more connected to her."

Rosalyn nodded in agreement. "I feel the same way. I didn't realize how much my work habits were affecting Mia, and I feel more motivated to spend more time with her and to check in with her more frequently on what she needs from me."

"That's fantastic," I affirmed, smiling warmly at them. "You both did an excellent job using the repair process. To stay on track, I want you to continue to do your daily check-ins with each other, and if an issue comes up, try using this repair process." Mia and Rosalyn left my office holding hands, a clear indication of progress in their relationship.

Having now equipped yourself with an abundant supply of tools to strengthen your emotional connection and build more robust emotional resilience within your relationship, it's time to shift our focus. In Part Three of this book, we're delving into enhancing and enriching the physical and sexual dimensions of your relationship.

# PART THREE
# SEXUAL INTIMACY—REKINDLING DESIRE

When I sat down to start writing this book, I assumed that writing the chapters about sexual intimacy would flow from my fingertips like water—quickly, naturally, effortlessly. The truth is I've really struggled to get all these thoughts down on paper. Part of this is because there's so much information to impart about different sexual techniques. I've already covered many of them in *Living an Orgasmic Life,* and there are hundreds of excellent resources including books, videos, apps, and online classes that provide detailed information about orgasms, sex, Tantra, kink, you name it. I will provide a detailed list of resources with some of my favorites at the end of the book.

I chose to focus on three critical components of sexual intimacy which are not discussed as frequently, and which form the basis for creating a lifetime of passionate intimacy. The first chapter forms the framework for creating a new paradigm of sex with practical tools and tips to enhance your sex life. The second and third chapters delve into your personal sexual preferences—exploring how your unique desires and tendencies shape what arouses you physically.

These chapters also examine the crucial emotional dimensions that transform physical acts into deeply intimate experiences.

What's critical for you to understand is that creating a lifetime of passionate intimacy is not just about technique or positions, it's really about learning how to create deep emotional intimacy with your partner. It is from that place of emotional safety where each of you feels truly seen that sexual intimacy flows. Fully opening yourself up sexually requires being incredibly vulnerable and trusting that you will not be judged for your wants, needs, and desires.

# 8

# REIGNITING SEXUAL INTIMACY

Communication is key. If you were to ask any sex therapist what's most important to maintain a healthy sex life, their answer would be open and honest communication. Without it, misunderstandings, unmet needs, and unspoken desires can create distance and resentment between partners.

Openly discussing your desires, boundaries, and sexual satisfaction helps build trust and emotional safety, which are essential for deep and fulfilling intimacy. When you feel safe to express what turns you on, what you enjoy, and what you need more (or less) of, you can create a sex life that is satisfying, playful, and deeply connected.

The good news is that if you have mastered the skills you learned in the first two parts of this book, you are already well equipped to have these important conversations about sex and intimacy. The same principles of active listening, expressing yourself clearly and directly, sharing vulnerably, and validating your partner's perspective apply just as much to discussions about your sex life as they do to any other topic in your relationship.

Unfortunately, even couples who have great communication skills will often have challenges talking about sex, which for many individuals is an uncomfortable and taboo subject. So, let's examine what some of the barriers are and identify ways you can overcome them. For a detailed exploration of why you might face difficulties related to sex, I encourage you to read Part One of my book, *Living an Orgasmic Life*, where I delve deeply into this topic.

**Case Study: Jennifer and Julian**

Jennifer and Julian were sitting in my office complaining about their sex life, or lack thereof.

Jennifer spoke first; her voice tinged with frustration. "We used to have such a passionate relationship, but lately it feels like we're just going through the motions. I don't know how to bring the spark back."

Julian nodded in agreement; his eyes fixed on the floor. "I love Jennifer, but I feel like we're disconnected in the bedroom. I'm not sure what she wants anymore."

I nodded, sensing the tension between them. "How long has this been going on?"

"About a year," Jennifer replied. "Ever since our second child was born."

"And have you two discussed this with each other before coming to see me?" I asked.

They exchanged a glance, looking slightly embarrassed.

"Not really," Julian admitted. "I mean, we've made comments here and there, but we've never sat down to have a real conversation about it."

"What's prevented you from having that conversation?" I asked gently.

Jennifer looked down at the floor for a moment and revealed, "I've never been comfortable talking about sex with anyone. Growing up, sex was a taboo subject in my home and community."

"That's understandable, Jennifer," I said softly. "Many people struggle with discussing sex openly due to their upbringing or cultural background. Julian, how about you?"

Julian shifted in his seat. "I guess I've been afraid of saying the wrong thing or hurting Jennifer's feelings. It's easier to just avoid the topic altogether."

I leaned forward, my expression compassionate. "It's completely normal to feel uncomfortable discussing sex, especially if you've never really done it before. But avoiding these conversations is often what leads to the disconnection you're experiencing now. What if we started small? Could you each share one thing you miss about your sex life from before?"

"I really miss how we used to make out on the couch at night," Jennifer said, looking up shyly. Julian nodded in agreement. "That was so much fun. I really miss how you used to come up behind me when I wasn't expecting it and give me a squeeze. I loved knowing that you wanted to touch my body," he said wistfully.

"That was a great start," I told them with a smile. "Now let's explore some of the reasons talking about sex is so hard for you."

## SHAME AROUND SEX

It's a tragedy that most human beings have so much shame around sex, especially since we are designed to experience pleasure. From the moment we leave the womb until social conditioning kicks in, we are free to explore and touch our bodies. Babies and toddlers love putting their toes in their mouth, coo when they are nursing, touch themselves all over, and freely express pleasure. Unfortunately, as we get older, we are compelled by our environment to rein in our pleasure-seeking impulses, especially those that are sexual in nature. Little ones naturally reach for their genitals, and when they do, are often subtly or overtly reprimanded. Thus begins the negative social conditioning around sex.

Although sexual shame isn't inherently linked to a specific gender, in my professional observation, women tend to feel it more acutely and have been conditioned to say "no" to sex. Normalizing the conversation about sex has been one of my professional goals for the last fifteen years. While I've seen some progress with more information available on social media platforms, as well as a plethora of podcasters and Instagram sex personalities, I've also noticed a concerning trend of increased shame and anxiety around sex and our bodies, especially among younger generations. A perfect example is the shift that's been happening in women's health club locker rooms, where private changing rooms are taking over the ubiquitous open locker rooms of the past. This change reflects a growing discomfort with nudity and our bodies, even in single-sex spaces.

Moreover, the conservative shift of the United States in 2025, the ever-increasing restrictions on sex education and women's autonomy over our bodies, and the reemergence of the religious right are moving us backward in terms of sexual liberation and acceptance. This shame and discomfort around our bodies and sexuality bleeds into our intimate relationships. Many couples struggle to openly discuss their desires, fantasies, and needs in the bedroom. The fear of judgment or rejection can be paralyzing, leading to a breakdown in communication, and ultimately, in sexual satisfaction.

## YOUR SEXUAL BLUEPRINT

For Jennifer and Julian, their individual experiences with shame were impacting their ability to connect intimately. As we continued our session, I guided them through exercises to help identify and challenge their internalized shame around sex.

"Jennifer, you mentioned that sex was a taboo subject in your home growing up. Can you tell me more about that?" I gently inquired.

Jennifer took a deep breath. "My parents never talked about sex. If anything remotely sexual came on TV, they'd change the channel or make us leave the room. In our church youth group, I was taught that sex was dirty, that touching yourself is a sin and would lead you to hell, and that sex in marriage is only for the man's pleasure."

I took a breath and spoke gently to Jennifer.

"These early experiences and messages form what we call your 'sexual blueprint.' It's the foundation upon which your attitudes and beliefs about sex are built. Understanding this blueprint is crucial because it often unconsciously influences your sexual behavior and communication as an adult."

Jennifer nodded slowly, her eyes widening with understanding. "I never thought about it that way before. I guess those early messages really stuck with me."

"What's important for you to realize, Jennifer, is that the feelings of shame that you are experiencing are not your fault. They were foisted upon you by others, your parents, your church, and your community. The good news is you can work to overcome them."

With that information, Jennifer's whole body relaxed. "What about you, Julian, what messages did you receive about sex growing up?"

Julian paused, considering the question. "Well, I didn't get much education about sex at home either. My dad would make crude jokes sometimes, but we never had any real conversations about it. I learned most of what I know from friends and, well, porn."

I nodded understandingly. "That's not uncommon. Many people, especially men, turn to pornography as a source of sexual education in the absence of open, honest discussions. However, porn often presents an unrealistic and sometimes harmful view of sex and relationships."

"Now that we've identified some of your sexual blueprints, I'm going to give you this sexual blueprint exercise as home play—the fun version of homework! Make sure to write down your answers. Then I want you to take some time to share your answers with each other. This is the first step towards overcoming your sexual shame."

## *Sexual Blueprint Exercise*

Think about your own childhood and what kind of messages you received about sex from your parents, other adults, and society. Reflect on the following questions. Write down any images that come to mind. Writing down what you notice gives your memory permission to open up and deliver more information about a particular incident or scene.

- Did you see your parents hold hands and touch each other? How often?
- Did your parents kiss in front of you?
- Were their kisses tender or perfunctory?
- Were you allowed to crawl into your parents' bed to cuddle?
- Did you ever see your parents or other adults naked? What were the circumstances?
- Did your parents make you hide your eyes if there was a romantic scene on TV?
- When did you first learn about sex? Where or from whom?
- Was there ever any discussion about sex in your family?
- Was sex discussed in any religious or cultural communities you belonged to?

- At what age do you remember first exploring your body and genitals and experiencing some sensation? Did you do this alone or with a sibling or friend?
- Were you ever afraid that you might get caught exploring or touching yourself? If you did have the experience of being caught, describe what happened and how it made you feel.

Now that you have a better understanding of your sexual blueprint, let's look at the impact it's had on your sex life.

- How does your sexual blueprint impact your adult sexual relationships?
- Did you previously notice that so many of the beliefs that you have about sex come from others?
- If you were to rid yourself of those false beliefs, how would that impact your sexuality?

Your sexual blueprint is key to understanding and changing your relationship with sex and intimacy.

## CREATING A SAFE SPACE FOR A CONVERSATION ABOUT YOUR SEXUAL RELATIONSHIP

Jennifer and Julian's story illustrates a universal truth: When we can't talk openly about sex, we can't transform our intimate experiences. The discomfort of these conversations becomes a wall between where we are and where we want to be. As we've discussed previously, emotional disconnection also becomes a barrier to intimacy.

But what if you could create a space that provides the opportunity for you both to be exquisitely present with each other, clear some of these emotional blocks, and drop into a safe place where these conversations can take place?

### *Exercise: Sacred Space Ritual—A Partner Practice*

(Included with permission from Skydancing USA's Timeless Loving Workshop)

This is one of the most powerful ways for you to connect with your partner when you're feeling disconnected or want to prepare for an intimate conversation about sex. The ritual helps create a container of safety and trust that makes vulnerability easier. In the world of Tantra, it is most often used as part of an intimate sexual experience. This is definitely a practice favored by my clients and one of the practices that they use on an ongoing basis.

Step 1: Choose a quiet time when you won't be interrupted. Turn off phones and other distractions. Create a comfortable environment on the bed or the floor with pillows, soft lighting, and perhaps gentle music. Optional: Light a candle to symbolize the sacred nature of your connection.

Step 2: Sit cross-legged on the ground or in chairs, facing each other with knees almost touching. Take a minute to close your eyes and feel your own body. Open your eyes and look at your partner's eyes with soft focus. Take a few deep breaths together, synchronizing your breathing if possible.

Step 3. Each of you place your hands together in a prayer position and gently bow to each other, acknowledging and thanking your partner for engaging in this ritual with you.

Step 4. With your hands, form an imaginary bubble around the two of you, ensuring it's sealed securely. This bubble represents a private space that includes only the two of you. It travels with you wherever you go—be it the hot tub, shower, or bedroom—and remains intact until you choose to pop it at the conclusion of your intimate time together.

Step 5. Take turns removing items from the bubble that will not be helpful for you. You may only take your own things out, not your partner's, and you are not allowed to discuss these items or question your partner about them. This is where we get rid of emotional congestion.

Examples include "distractions," "not being focused," "being tired," "being upset about our fight this morning," "the kids waking up," "your family," and so on. Keep on going until each of you feels complete.

Step 6. Now take turns bringing into the bubble the qualities and experiences you want, such as "connection," "love," "sexiness," "playfulness," "vulnerability," "honesty," and so on.

Step 7. Take turns giving each other three compliments, stating specifically what you appreciate about your partner. You can complement his/her physical attributes ("I love how your eyes twinkle when I look into them"), other qualities ("You have such a big heart"), or specific actions ("It was so great how you helped our neighbors shovel their snow"). The more specific you are, the more solidly the appreciation will land.

Step 8. In the next step, you will take turns stating your desires, fears, and boundaries for whatever activity you may be engaging in.

For the purposes of a communication exercise around sex, you would state desires, fears, and boundaries around your communication. For example:

"My desire is to be vulnerable and authentic."

"My fear is that I might hurt your feelings, and you might shut down."

"My boundary is that I do not want to talk about specific incidents in the past."

If you are creating sacred space as part of an intimate sexual experience, then your desires, fears and boundaries might sound like this:

"My desire is that we touch each other for thirty minutes before having sex."

"My fear is that you might want to go faster than I do and I won't be able to find my voice to slow things down."

"My boundary is no 'doggie style.'"

When stating your desires, fears, and boundaries, be sure that you are only talking about your own desires and not projecting on your partner. It's fine to say: "My desire is that you touch me all over my body with a feather." It's not okay to say: "My desire is that you don't touch me the horrible way you touched me last time we had sex."

Most of us find it a bit challenging to set boundaries, and often it is even more so with an intimate partner. Some people feel uncomfortable talking about what's okay and not okay. Others aren't even aware they have boundaries or only become aware when a boundary is crossed. But setting boundaries with your partner is important for many reasons, and this exercise gives you the opportunity to practice that skill. You can set boundaries about time, parts of your body you don't want touched, or activities you don't want to engage in.

Step 9. Once the activity or conversation wraps up, regroup, and sitting face-to-face in your bubble, bow to each other and then deliberately raise your fingers to pop the imaginary bubble.

## *How Do You Like to be Loved? An Intimate Communication Exercise*

This practice, which happens within the sacred space you just created, will help you and your partner understand each other's needs and desires around love and sex.

- Sit across from each other and decide who will begin.
- Partner 1 sets a timer for three minutes and poses the first question to Partner 2: "How do you like to be loved?" Partner 2 gives a brief response, such as, "I feel loved when you massage my feet."
- Partner 1 acknowledges with a 'thank you' and then repeats the same question, "How do you like to be loved?" This exchange continues until the timer signals the end of the three minutes.
- Next, Partner 1 follows the same procedure for the next two questions: "How can I love you more?" and "What holds you back sexually?"
- Then switch and repeat the exercise with Partner 2 asking the questions.

Once you've both finished, take a moment to talk over and reflect on your responses without any shame or judgment towards yourself or your partner. Remain open-minded and observe if either of you shared any surprising information. This is a chance to explore in a safe environment, so feel free to ask your partner questions about their answers. Pay attention to what you learn from this discussion.

Common Pitfalls:

This practice is often more challenging than it seems because it requires each of you to identify your wants and needs and clearly communicate them.

- Answering the same question repeatedly gives you the opportunity for deeper reflection. If you find yourself getting stuck, try closing your eyes and continue to answer the questions. State the first thing that comes to mind and don't overthink it.
- Avoid editing your answers so as not to upset your partner. This is an opportunity for total vulnerability and authenticity.
- Remember there are many ways in which we can feel loved (physical, emotional, acts of service, and more). Think about what's really important for you, not what you think your partner wants to hear.
- It's important to be able to tell your partner how they can love you more. Many of my couples struggle with this question, fearing that they are hurting their partner. Remember, even though you might feel totally loved and taken care of, there's almost always something else that would make you feel more loved. This is a golden opportunity to express that desire.
- Some couples find it difficult to articulate what holds them back sexually because they've never really examined their own barriers. Take time to consider what prevents you from fully expressing yourself sexually—it could be body image issues, past trauma, fear of judgment, or simply lack of knowledge about what you enjoy.

When I first introduced this exercise to Jennifer and Julian in our next session, they were hesitant but willing to try. Jennifer discovered that she felt most loved when Julian took time to connect with her emotionally before any physical intimacy began. "I need to feel seen and heard," she explained. "When we jump straight into physical touch without talking first, I feel like an object rather than a person."

Julian was surprised by his own responses. "I realized I feel most loved when Jennifer initiates touch," he admitted. "I always thought I was supposed to be the one making the first move, but actually, when she reaches for me, it makes me feel desired."

"I love that you're both learning more about what your needs and desires are and how to share that with each other," I said. "But Julian, you just raised an important subject about unexpressed expectations and pressure that you have around initiating sex. Let's dive more into that topic!"

## THE INITIATION GAME

How and by whom sex is initiated is one of couples' most common pain points. If you could sit in my office for a month and listen to the secret stories of couples, you would soon hear the same two refrains echoing through every retelling of sexual frustration: (1) "He doesn't know how to turn me on" and (2) "She never initiates." The forms these complaints take are as varied as the couples themselves, but the underlying emotional chords of disappointment, rejection, and resentment are always familiar.

Unfortunately, these patterns are rarely voiced until they have turned into years of frustration and resentment, and then the partners land in my office at the end of their rope.

"Jennifer, in this last exercise, you said that one of the things that holds you back sexually is that you don't like the way Julian initiates sex. Can you talk more about that?"

Jennifer started talking, hesitantly at first until Julian nodded his head, reassuring her that he wanted to hear her concerns.

"Usually it's late at night, in bed, and he reaches over and starts rubbing my leg. That's the signal that he wants sex."

“What happens next?” I asked.

“If I don’t say no or turn the other way, his hand quickly finds my vagina, and he starts rubbing my clit hard. If he thinks I’m enjoying it (which I’m not), he might go down on me for two minutes and then stick his penis in.”

“And how does that make you feel?” I gently pried. “Terrible, I feel like a piece of meat just there for his pleasure and satisfaction.”

This is a far too common refrain that I hear from women in my practice. There are many variations on it, each describing a moment when desire feels imposed rather than invited: “When he comes up behind me while I'm washing dishes and presses against me," or "When he starts rubbing my shoulders while I'm working at my laptop," or "When he hugs me longer than usual while I'm getting ready in the morning."

These are all signals that women have learned to recognize as sexual overtures that bypass their emotional needs. The problem is that there is often misinterpretation around these actions. Many of these actions (touching, hugging) are what women say they want more of. The line between welcome affection and unwanted advance seems impossibly thin, leaving both partners walking a tightrope of confusion.

“How would you like Julian to initiate sex?” I asked.

“I want him to romance me —to take me out to a nice dinner that I didn’t have to plan, put his phone away, and ask about my day. I need to feel closer to him, to feel like he sees me as a person, not just a sex object.”

“So, it sounds like you need more of an emotional connection with Julian before wanting sex. What about the physical part of initiation?”

"I want things to move much slower. I want to make out first, I want him to touch me slowly, to caress my hair and face—to tell me that I'm beautiful and he loves me."

I turned to Julian. "How does it feel to hear Jennifer's perspective on initiating sex?"

Honestly, it's hard to hear, but I'm glad she's telling me. I had no idea she felt that way. I thought I was being romantic and spontaneous by touching her." He paused, running his hand through his hair. "I guess I've been doing what I thought worked, but I never actually asked her what she wanted."

"Julian, your intentions were good, but your approach wasn't meeting Jennifer's needs," I explained. "This is exactly why communication is so crucial. Now, Jennifer, I want to ask you something. When Julian initiates in ways that don't work for you, what do you typically do?"

Jennifer shifted uncomfortably. "I usually just go along with it, or else I find an excuse to say no. I've never actually told him what I need."

"And Julian, when Jennifer says no or seems uninterested, how do you interpret that?"

"I feel rejected," he admitted. "I start thinking she doesn't find me attractive anymore, or that she doesn't want me. Then I am more and more afraid to initiate sex."

"I hear this all the time," I reassured him. "Rejection always hurts; it hits a very deep place inside of us that makes us feel not good enough and that we're not measuring up to what society expects of us."

Men have their own burdens around initiating sex, and like Julian, often find themselves locked into the role of perpetual initiator. They are also always balancing the emotional calculus of risk and rejection, ranging from a gentle "not now honey, I'm tired tonight," to a more exasperated sigh that is far more wounding. Over the years, the rejection and resentment pile up, leaving many men feeling they are not wanted. The fact that their partner rarely, if ever, initiates sex exacerbates the problem and the feeling of not being desired.

Although this same pattern repeats itself in the overwhelming majority of long-term relationships, it's important not to cast any blame here. The truth is that no one actually taught us how to have sex or how to initiate sex. So, let's start with the basics.

## TOUCH 101

Let me be candid: When it comes to initiating sex, most of us fumble in the dark. We've mastered the basics—the reassuring squeeze of hands, the comfort of an embrace, the warmth of bodies curled together on the couch. But that crucial transition from affection to arousal? That's where even the most loving partners often resort to clumsy, predictable moves that miss their mark entirely.

I witness this in my office constantly; light rubbing of the arm, using fingernails to gently scratch the same area of the body over and over again. Frequently, when I ask someone to show me how they touch their partner in a sensual way, the only response I get is a vacant stare. Again, this is not your fault! No one taught you how to touch your partner.

Touch is the first of our senses that develops in utero, and as such, touch is the first language we learn. Soft, gentle touch releases oxytocin into the bloodstream, creating trust. That trust in turn reduces cortisol, the stress hormone. Decreasing cortisol levels allows your body to relax, which is a critical component of building up arousal, especially for women.

We think that the process of touching a partner is quite straightforward, but in fact, there is a whole relationship dynamic involved in touch. Betty Martin, author and creator of the Wheel of Consent, has created a whole body of work around touch. In her workshops, she teaches a process of giving and receiving touch that allows each partner to consider their boundaries, what they are willing to give, what they are willing to receive, how they want to be touched by their partner, and how they want to touch their partner.

In Martin's game, the role of "taking" contains a principle of touch that will completely change your experience of pleasure. The principle is touching for your own pleasure. The principle is a mindset shift, meaning you will start to look at the whole arena of touch from a different perspective than the one to which you are accustomed.

To illustrate this, let's drop in on my touch session with Jennifer and Julian.

"Julian, will you show me how you would touch Jennifer's arm if you wanted to initiate sex?"

Julian looked at me quizzically and then started to lightly rub his fingertips up and down a five-inch portion of the outside of Jennifer's arm.

"Jennifer, on a scale of one to ten, how would you rate Julian's touch in terms of how much pleasure you received from it?"

Jennifer replied, "I would give it about a four." This is a fairly typical response when we do this exercise.

"Now, Julian, when you were touching Jennifer, what were you thinking about? Where did you put your attention?" I gently asked.

Julian said, "I was looking at her face trying to see if she liked what I was doing."

"Exactly," I replied, "you really wanted to make it feel pleasurable for her, but how did it feel for you?"

Julian looked at me quizzically, "I don't really know, I wasn't thinking about that."

A knowing smile crossed my face.

"Let's try this exercise again, and this time, Julian, you're going to close your eyes and touch Jennifer's arm in a way that feels pleasurable for you. I don't want you to be concerned about how it feels for her right now, but I do want you to really focus on the sensation in your hand...think about using Jennifer's arm to make your whole hand feel good. You might also try slowing down and using your whole hand, not just your fingertips."

Julian followed my instructions, slowed down his touch, and began to gently touch and explore Jennifer's arm. I also advised him to take a few deep breaths. After a few minutes, I could see them both visibly relax, and a little smile emerged on Jennifer's lips.

"Jennifer," I asked, "how would you rate Julian's touch now?"

Jennifer gave a warm smile, "Oh, that felt amazing; I would give it a nine." Julian looked up in surprise.

"What felt different for you?" I prodded.

"I felt like Julian was actually paying attention, it just felt much more intentional," Jennifer explained.

"Great!" I exclaimed. "And Julian, what was that experience like for you?"

"I really enjoyed touching Jennifer's arm. It felt so soft on my fingertips, and she didn't freeze up or pull away like she normally does. I could have continued that for longer!" We all laughed.

"Perfect," I exclaimed. "I'm teaching you a very important touch concept called 'touching for your own pleasure.' It will completely transform the way you think about touching your partner."

## Touching for Your Own Pleasure

Generally, when we touch our partners, we are not doing it for our own pleasure and sensation. You touch your partner the way you think they want to be touched. If you are really attuned to your partner, you might ask them for feedback about your touch and then make an adjustment based on their response.

On the other hand, touching for your own pleasure means that you touch your partner in a way that feels really pleasurable to you, focusing specifically on the sensations in your hands or whatever other body part you are using for touch (perhaps your mouth, tongue, or breasts). Touching for your own pleasure is a much more conscious way of touching your partner which brings more presence into the encounter.

When you touch your partner in a way that brings you pleasure, it amplifies their pleasure as well. Your enjoyment heightens their arousal, which in turn boosts their enjoyment of your touch. This, in turn, enhances your own excitement, forming a pleasure circuit between the two of you.

I can't begin to emphasize enough how important it is to learn and practice this concept as it will have a tremendous impact on your sex life. This is particularly true for both women and men around giving oral sex. When you stop worrying about performing for your partner and focus on your own pleasure and enjoyment (with of course feedback from your partner if something doesn't feel pleasurable), it will completely transform your experience. Thinking about using your partner's body to make your body feel great shifts touching your partner from being a "job" to a delicious feast for your senses.

However, it's important to note that touching for your own pleasure doesn't mean ignoring your partner's comfort or boundaries. It's about finding the intersection where your pleasure and their comfort meet. This requires ongoing communication and awareness.

## The Four Different Types of Touch

A common obstacle for couples is not realizing that there are various ways to touch your partner that can spark intimacy and trigger the path to arousal. In teaching different ways to touch, I like to refer to the four elements: earth, water, air, fire.

*Earth Touch*: Earth touch is grounding touch. It creates comfort and safety for your partner. Earth touch is slow, still, and often involves some pressure: a long melting hug, pressing your hands down on your partner's shoulders, coming behind them and wrapping your arms around their chest, pulling them into you tightly by their hips or butt, not for the purpose of making genital contact, but for creating slow, safe connection.

Earth touch is also very useful when you first touch your partner's genitals; a firm hand over the pussy or cock for thirty seconds is very grounding and supportive. It says, "I'm here and you're safe." Earth touch is often a great way to initiate a sexual encounter.

*Water Touch:* Water touch is flowing, sensual touch. It is designed to awaken the senses without necessarily leading to sex. This touch builds anticipation and desire.

Water touch is light touch, gentle caresses, stroking the hair and face. Flowing touch means that there are long, full strokes, using your entire hand including the palm (such as stroking up the entire arm to the shoulder). Water touch can also involve using fingertips and light, gentle massage. The focus is generally on non-erogenous zones.

*Air Touch:* Air touch is extremely light, airy, teasing touch. It's often used to build arousal and give your partner a sense of anticipation that might even result in gooseflesh, aka "chill bumps."

It's a touch that barely connects with your partner's skin—you might be touching just the hairs on their arm. Air touch can also mean energetic touch so that you're "touching" the aura or energetic space around your partner (3 to 6 inches away from their skin). Air touch may also involve blowing cool air or hot air on your partner's skin, or into their ears.

*Fire Touch:* Fire touch is a more passionate, erotic touch. It signals to your partner that you desire and hunger for them. It's more of an animalistic type of touch, typically leading to more sexual exploration.

Fire touch includes scratching, biting, hair pulling, and smacking your partner on the butt. It also includes compression touch. For example, pulling your partner close to you, pressing your hands into their arms, pulling their hips into you, or pressing your whole body against them.

## *Touch Exercise:*

1. Partner 1 sets a 90-second timer and begins touching Partner 2 with Earth Touch. Partner 2 then touches Partner 1 with Earth Touch for 90-seconds. Then share with each other what that felt like and what you each liked or didn't like.
2. Repeat this same process for Water Touch, Air Touch, and Fire Touch.

Doing this touch exercise will help you understand better what type of touch you like or don't like. Go into this with an open mind, and don't judge yourself or your partner. Touch is a very individual experience, and it can change from day to day. Most importantly it will give you some language to ask for what you want. It will also help you to better understand your own individual arousal pathway, which we will spend more time on in the next chapter.

Also, I know you're hoping that I'm going to give you the secret formula for combining all these touches so that it will work perfectly every time. Spoiler alert: Sex and touch is an art, not a science. What works for one person, may be different than what works for another. It can also change from day to day. For example, I really love it when Daren initiates with soft, sensual touch. Other times I just want him to throw me up against the wall and start ravishing me.

When Jennifer and Julian did this, they learned that Jennifer preferred to start with Earth touch—she loved feeling grounded and safe before moving into more sensual territory. "The firm pressure on my shoulders made me feel like you were really present with me," she told Julian. "It helped me relax instead of feeling like you were just trying to get somewhere quickly."

Julian discovered he was drawn to Fire touch but realized it was too intense as an opener for Jennifer. "I love the passionate energy of it," he explained, "but I can see now why it might feel overwhelming if we haven't built up to it."

What surprised them both was how much they enjoyed the Air touch. "I never realized how sensitive I am to that barely-there touching," Jennifer admitted with a blush. "It made me want more."

In the next chapter we're going to explore women's and men's arousal pathways and sexual styles in more detail. But I do want you to remember that initiating sex is not just about the physical act—it's also about creating the right emotional environment where desire can flow. The emotional connection that we've been talking about in the first two parts of this book forms the foundation for successful physical intimacy. When the members of a couple each feel emotionally connected, trusted, and valued by their partner, they are much more likely to be open to sexual connection.

# 9
# CREATING A NEW PARADIGM FOR SEX

What was your sex education like? If you are like most people, the answer would be "not much." If you were lucky, you had a sex education class in school where you learned a little about anatomy and reproduction. But most of us learned how to have sex by watching movies and porn, or by trial and error. We learned a paint by numbers approach: Insert penis into vagina, race to climax, which will magically happen simultaneously, and cue the fireworks. We learned a model where "real sex" means penetration and success means orgasm.

How well is that approach serving you now? If it was working, you likely wouldn't be reading this book! That model is beyond broken and leaves out so many possibilities for what sex can be with your partner. It's time to create a new paradigm—one based in pleasure, curiosity, connection, and embodiment.

This chapter is about busting myths and helping you create a new paradigm for your sex life. We'll explore the key differences between male and female arousal and explore why it's so important for women to slow things down. We'll redefine what sex means (it's not just penis in vagina), eliminate the focus on goals, and dive into the anatomy of arousal—because knowing your way around a vulva or a penis is foundational, not optional.

## UNDERSTAND THE DIFFERENCE BETWEEN WOMEN'S AND MEN'S AROUSAL

In 1992, John Grey wrote the best-selling book *Men are from Mars, Women are from Venus*. In this book, he explains how men and women often have fundamentally different communication styles, emotional needs, and coping strategies. There's only one important piece he left out—-we also have vastly different sexual arousal pathways, which creates another significant pain point for couples around sex.

Here's the Cliff Notes version: Men are like microwave popcorn; women are like a cake baked in an oven.

Meet my clients Monica and Morgan. They have been married for five years and came to a retreat because sex had become less and less frequent and they wanted to address it before it became a bigger problem.

Morgan had a very common complaint, "When Morgan wants to have sex, he grabs my boobs, and it's such a turnoff," she told me.

"I just want to show her some love," Morgan said.

"I completely understand that, Morgan, and I am sure you're confused why that doesn't turn Monica on. I bet if she grabbed your cock, you'd be ready to go, right?" He nodded in agreement.

"This is a great time for us to talk about the differences between men's arousal and women's arousal, and it all has to do with our anatomy." I said.

## SAME PARTS, ARRANGED DIFFERENTLY

Believe it or not, male and female genitals are made from the exact same genetic tissues. In the early weeks of development in the womb, every embryo starts with the same basic set of genital parts. It's hormones—specifically testosterone—that influence how those parts eventually take shape.

That means the penis and the clitoris. Same tissue, different design. The scrotum and the labia? Also cut from the same cloth. Even deep inside, the ovaries and the testes are anatomical siblings, both responsible for producing sex hormones and reproductive cells.

However, the size and location of our external genitals are vastly different, and these differences significantly impact our arousal pathway.

"Morgan, since you came out of the womb, you have worn your arousal equipment (penis and scrotum) on the outside of your body, where it's been very available and easy for you to touch and make contact with, and you touched yourself as a baby and as a child, all the time. Even to pee, you had your hand on your penis, and it might even have felt good!" Morgan laughed at this.

"And as you grew into adolescence and your hormones started to surge, you started to experience more arousal and erections, both voluntary when you masturbated as well as involuntary."

"Having a hard-on in school out of the blue was the worst!" Morgan sheepishly acknowledged.

"I know. It's so hard for adolescent boys," I empathically responded. "Your penis, at a very early age, got acclimated to responding to stimuli—even just from having it constantly be touched by underwear and pants. So, it makes perfect sense that if Monica were to reach out and grab your penis, or even just give you a sexy look, you'll get hard and be ready for sex."

Morgan said, "It doesn't take much for me to get hard; even talking about this is kind of exciting for me."

I laughed. "This is why men assume that a woman's body will have the exact same reaction when their genitals (including nipples and vulva) are touched," I explained.

"Now let's consider female anatomy. Unlike men, 90 percent of a woman's arousal equipment (clitoris, labia, G-spot) are worn on the inside of our body. The only external part of our clitoris is the head and part of the shaft, and even that is covered by the clitoral hood, which shields it from exposure. Unlike the penis, the clitoris is not easy to access for a child, it is not constantly being exposed to stimuli, and you do not hold it or even touch it when you go to pee," I explained.

Monica said, "I didn't even find my clitoris until high school, and was still too afraid to touch myself, given what I was told at religious school."

"I'm so sorry," I sighed. "When girls are going through puberty, unlike boys, there's really no anatomical signal around arousal. It's not like they see a hot boy, feel their clitoris getting engorged, and go to the bathroom to start masturbating," I explained. They both giggled at this.

"But let's be clear. Women's bodies have a vast array of nerves and erectile tissue that form our arousal network from our nipples all the way deep into our vulva and vagina. It's just that in order to get our arousal network going, we have to create a different pathway."

"Morgan, you're like microwave popcorn," I explained. "Put in the right input—visual stimulation, direct touch—and boom, you're ready in a minute. Your arousal is external, visible, and quick to respond."

Morgan nodded, understanding dawning on his face.

"Monica, on the other hand, is like a cake baking in an oven. Her arousal needs preheating, careful preparation, and time to rise. It's an inside-out process rather than an outside-in one."

Monica nodded enthusiastically. "That's exactly how it feels! When Morgan just grabs my breasts out of nowhere, it's like he's trying to frost a cake that hasn't even gone into the oven yet."

"Precisely," I said. "For women, arousal typically begins in the brain, not the genitals. The brain is actually your largest sex organ, Monica. Before your body can respond, your mind needs to shift into a sexual space."

"So, what does that mean for us?" Morgan asked, leaning forward with genuine curiosity.

"It means that you need to slow everything down. Think about foreplay starting way before you touch Monica," I explained. "Send her a sexy text in the morning or even the day before. Give her brain some time to register that an erotic date is on the table. And when you do initiate physical contact, be sure that you really spend plenty of time touching the non-erogenous parts of her body first."

"Monica's arousal needs a gradual build-up that engages her mind first, then slowly works through her body to her genitals. Remember it's a journey, not a destination," I explained.

Monica nodded. "That makes so much sense. When Morgan just goes straight for my breasts or between my legs, I feel like I'm being rushed to the finish line of a race I haven't even started."

"I know this might surprise you," I added, "but most women need a minimum of thirty to forty-five minutes of foreplay—touching, kissing, oral sex, dirty words—before their body is ready for penetration."

Both Morgan and Monica looked shocked at this number.

"Thirty minutes?" Morgan said, his eyes widening. "I had no idea. I thought maybe five or ten minutes was plenty."

"And that's completely normal, Morgan. Nobody ever taught you this, and most couples never learn about these fundamental differences," I reassured him. "The good news is that once you understand how Monica's body works, you can become an incredible lover for her."

Monica squeezed Morgan's hand. "I never knew how to explain this to you before. I thought something was wrong with me because I couldn't just flip a switch like you could."

"Nothing is wrong with either of you," I reassured them. "You just have different operating systems. The key is learning how to sync them up."

## SLOW DOWN

As you just witnessed in Monica and Morgan's session, one of the common pain points for couples is rushing into sexual intercourse, well before the female partner is ready. This creates a cascade of problems for women that will negatively impact your sex life.

- Insufficient arousal and lubrication of the vagina, making sex uncomfortable and even painful.
- Not feeling turned on and simply going through the motions creates a condition where sex is "okay" but not great, causing your partner to lose their desire for sex.
- Feeling like your partner is mis-attuned to your body, desire, and pleasure, again decreasing desire for more sex.

- Challenges getting to orgasm and/or not being able to experience deep intense orgasms that occur when the body is extremely aroused and stimulated in the right places and at the right time.
- Service or obligation sex for your partner's pleasure but not for yours.

Slowing down is one of the most powerful ways to mitigate all these challenges. Slowing down allows you to make contact with your body, your sensations, and your pleasure. When you slow down, look into each other's eyes, and focus on your connection, your bodies start to resonate in much the same way as two tuning forks set to the same note. You will start matching each other's breathing, and your movements will begin to flow and synchronize.

Remember that sex is an art form, not a science, and great sex means following the rhythm of your desires, body, and sensations. This cannot happen if you're on automatic and "going through the motions" or if one or both of you are in a hurry to have an orgasm and get it over with.

Slowing down allows you to:

- Become more present and aware of your body, sensations, and partner
- Build sexual energy slowly and create erotic tension
- Create resonance with your partner, enhancing connection and intimacy
- Have access to more of your pleasure centers, many of which need time to become activated

## REDEFINING SEX

I ask all my couples this question: "How do you define sex?" Ninety percent of them respond with the answer "sexual intercourse."

Therein lies one of the greatest problems when it comes to creating a great sex life, and also one of the easiest solutions.

It makes total sense that we all define sex as penetration, or as we like to call it in the sex therapy world, PIV (Penis in Vagina) sex. This is what we've learned and generally see in movies, TV, and porn.

But this is an incredibly narrow definition, and one that puts a tremendous amount of pressure on both you and your partner. What if we were to redefine sex as any activity that creates an erotic feeling or connection, regardless of whether physical contact is involved? If you're feeling dubious that sex can happen without physical contact, what happens when you have "phone sex" or "video sex"? Does arousal occur in your body? Are you always touching yourself, or sometimes, is just hearing your partner talking dirty to you a turn-on?

With this type of expanded definition of sex, the possibilities are limitless. Sex can become lying naked with each other and kissing, having a high school (first base) make out session on the couch, giving each other a sensual massage, telling each other what you'd like to do to them or what you'd like them to do to you, tying your partner up and teasing them with a feather, receiving a G-spot massage or prostate massage...the list goes on and on.

What's so powerful about this expanded definition of sex is that it relieves the pressure to perform for both women and men, opening a world of erotic potential for your sex life. When we take the goal orientation of penetration and orgasm off the table, you will be able to relax more, be more present with your partner, and be more in your experience of your pleasure. It allows you to enjoy the journey and not be concerned about the destination.

Expanding the definition is also very helpful for couples dealing with physical challenges and sexual dysfunction, as well as changes that happen to aging bodies.

Take my clients Alex and Jamie. When they first came to see me, Alex was dealing with erectile dysfunction that had developed after a stressful period at work. “Every time we start fooling around, all I can think about is whether I'll be able to get hard enough for intercourse,” he admitted. “And then, of course, I can't.”

Jamie nodded. “And then I feel rejected, like I'm not attractive enough to turn him on.”

“What if,” I suggested, “for the next month, you agree that intercourse is completely off the table? What if you explored all the other ways you can give each other pleasure?”

Alex took a deep breath; “That sounds so good to me,” he said. “I just want to be able to give Jamie pleasure and make her feel loved.”

Jamie squeezed Alex’s hand, and I saw his whole body relax. When Jamie and Alex came back to see me a few weeks later, they were thrilled to report that they were having great sexual experiences, they had learned a lot about each other’s bodies, and Jamie was even able to get an erection without trying.

## Lose the Goal Orientation

One of the reasons that women struggle with orgasms and men have erection issues (either struggling to keep one or ejaculating too quickly) is the performance pressure around sex. It’s been hardwired into our brains that successful sex ends in mind-blowing orgasms for both you and your partner.

Think about the pressure on both ends: For women, there’s pressure to get to orgasm quickly—so many women feel like they are taking too much time to orgasm, especially during oral sex. The result for many women is not being able to achieve orgasm, or as a last resort, faking orgasm. There are myriad reasons why women put this pressure on themselves.

- The unrealistic portrayal of orgasm in the media. How many times have you seen a man go down on a woman and she orgasms within a minute!
- Concern about bruising their partner's ego.
- Believing that their partner doesn't like how their pussy looks, feels, or tastes.
- They are not enjoying the experience so just want to get it over quickly.
- Too much attention on their body makes them uncomfortable.

For men, there is palpable pressure to ensure their partner reaches orgasm, to achieve and sustain an erection, to engage in penetration for as long as necessary for their partner to fully enjoy the experience, and to avoid ejaculating prematurely. For many men, "succeeding" in sex is deeply intertwined with their sense of masculinity, so any perceived shortcomings can feel like a profound failure.

When your mind fixates on reaching a specific outcome during sex, you're essentially splitting your attention—one part of you is engaged in the physical experience, while the other monitors your "progress." This mental multitasking disconnects you from both your partner's responses and your own body's signals. The pleasure that should naturally flow becomes interrupted by thoughts of "Am I doing this right?" or "Are we getting there yet?" The more you worry about performance, the less you can surrender to sensation, and the more difficult relaxation—the very foundation of any fulfilling sexual connection—becomes.

This is particularly important to understand for women who struggle with reaching orgasm and men dealing with early ejaculation challenges. For women, being in your head takes you out of the place of surrender and high arousal that you need to reach orgasm. Men with early ejaculation and anxiety struggle with noticing their body's arousal signals, so they quickly move from a

"3" on the arousal scale to an "9," which is past the point of no return.

## Put It on the Damn Calendar

Here's the deal. Life is busy, and schedules are crazy between work, kids, caregiving for older parents, and getting the dog to the vet. But if you look at your calendar, I imagine that you are going to see many outside activities scheduled: dinner with friends, a kid's baseball game, work functions. These events are on your calendar, so (1) you remember to attend and (2) each occasion is important to you—or it wouldn't make it onto your calendar. But what's not on your calendar is your weekly sexy time with your partner.

I can already hear the resistance; "Scheduling sex makes it feel like work," "Scheduling sex isn't spontaneous," "Scheduling sex feels like a lot of pressure." I've heard it all from my clients.

I know that scheduling sex seems the opposite of everything sexy, but I promise you that doing this will have a very positive impact on your sex life. When you schedule sex (as we have redefined it), you are making a bold statement; your relationship and your sex life are actually important priorities. Rather than sex becoming the last thing on your very long to-do list, it goes right to the top.

How you schedule it is entirely up to you and what works best in your life. Some of my clients have a regular day (for example, Saturday mornings). Daren and I usually sit down at the beginning of the week, look at our schedules, and then determine what would be the best day and hours for sexy time. For this process to be successful, you need to be very serious about scheduling it and not let the date continually "slip" because other more important priorities arise. Unless you're really injured or not feeling well, you can still cuddle up with your partner and have a little bit of bonding time as a couple—a gentle massage, some intimate talk time—anything to maintain the intimacy and connection you're creating with each other.

Let's address the biggest elephant in the room—the belief that sex *should* be spontaneous. When was the last time that you had great spontaneous sex? My guess is it was either when you were on vacation or back in the beginning of your relationship, when new relationship hormones were surging. How much do you really enjoy twenty minutes (if you're lucky) of "spontaneous sex" at the end of the night when you're already exhausted and getting into bed struggling to keep your eyes open? Does that kind of spontaneous sex create more or less desire inside of you?

Unlike spontaneous sex, when you schedule sex, it allows you to have more time and spaciousness for arousal and connection to build and for erotic exploration to occur. And you'll quickly find that when sex becomes more exciting, enjoyable, and intimate, you're going to want to have more of it, some of which will even be spontaneous. I have a favorite saying: "*Good sex begets more good sex*"—and the opposite is also true.

Speaking about calendars, I have a very special gift for you: A Couples Connection Calendar which you can download at https://www.passionateintimacyretreats.com/go-deeper/ . It's filled with daily invitations—some sweet, some spicy—to help you and your partner rebuild erotic energy and emotional closeness. These brief, real-world practices are designed to melt resistance, awaken desire, and remind you that intimacy can be fun again.

## ANATOMY OF THE VULVA AND THE PENIS

Going back to the terrible sex education that we all received, I would be remiss if I did not give you at least a broad overview of female and male anatomy, because I am continually shocked at how little my clients know about the anatomy of their own and their partner's sexual parts. I also want to offer a caveat here—the following is in no way comprehensive, and there are some incredible books and resources that go into much more detail (more on this at the end of the book). However, to really be able to experience high levels of arousal and pleasure, you must learn your way around each other's genitals and understand how arousal happens.

Let's start with the vulva, which is the main female genitalia, containing the labia (inner and outer lips), clitoral hood, clitoris, vagina, cervix, and the perineal and urethral sponges.

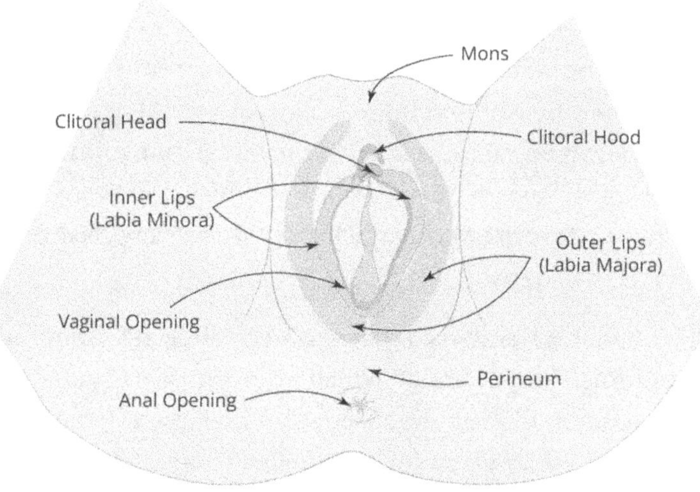


**External Genitalia (Vulva)**

**1. Mons Pubis**

A fatty pad of tissue over the pubic bone that cushions and protects the pelvic area. It becomes covered in pubic hair after puberty.

**2. Labia Majora (Outer Lips)**

Two outer folds of skin that protect the inner structures of the vulva.

They contain sweat and oil glands and are sensitive to touch and pressure.

**3. Labia Minora (Inner Lips)**

Thin, hairless folds located inside the labia majora. They protect the vaginal and urethral openings and swell with blood during arousal, increasing sensitivity.

**4. Clitoris**

A highly sensitive organ with both external and internal parts. The visible tip (glans) contains thousands of nerve endings, making it the primary source of female sexual pleasure. The internal parts (shaft, crura, and bulbs) fill with blood during arousal.

**5. Clitoral Hood (Prepuce)**

A small fold of skin that covers and protects the clitoral glans, similar to the foreskin on the penis.

**6. Urethral Opening**

The small opening just below the clitoris that carries urine from the bladder to the outside of the body.

**7. Vaginal Opening (Introitus)**

The entrance to the vagina, located below the urethral opening. It's surrounded by sensitive tissue and may be partially covered by a thin membrane called the hymen.

**8. Vestibular Bulbs**

Two elongated masses of erectile tissue located on either side of the vaginal opening. They swell during arousal, tightening the vaginal entrance and enhancing sensation.

**9. Bartholin's Glands (Greater Vestibular Glands)**

Two small glands on either side of the vaginal opening that secrete a lubricating fluid during arousal.

**10. Perineum**

The area of skin and muscle between the vaginal opening and the anus. It's sensitive and can contract rhythmically during orgasm.

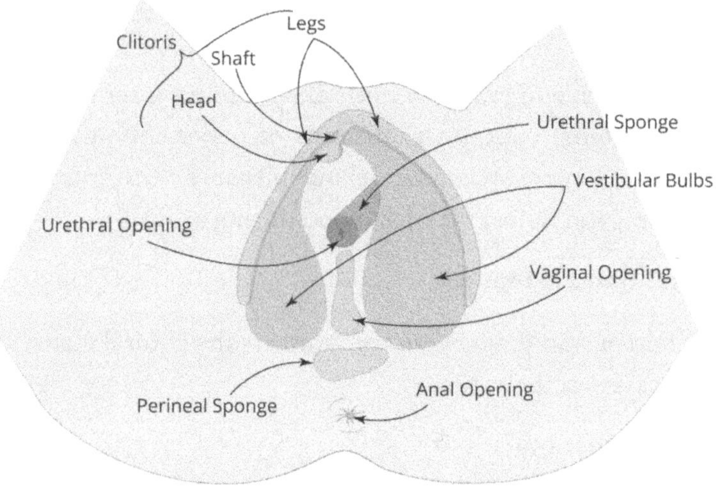


**Internal Genitalia (excluding uterus and ovaries)**

**1. Vagina**

A muscular, elastic canal that extends from the vaginal opening to the cervix. It receives the penis during intercourse, allows menstrual flow to exit, and serves as the birth canal.

**2. Clitoral Crura and Vestibular Bulbs (Internal Portions of Clitoris)**

The internal "legs" of the clitoris extend deep along the sides of the vaginal canal. Together with the bulbs, they form part of the internal erectile network that expands during arousal.

**3. Urethral Sponge (G-Spot Area)**

A spongy area located along the front vaginal wall surrounding the urethra. It contains erectile tissue and contributes to sexual pleasure and orgasmic response.

**4. Perineal Sponge**

Located between the vagina and rectum, this sponge-like tissue also engorges during arousal and adds to vaginal sensitivity.

**5. Cervix**

The **cervix** is the lower part of the uterus that connects to the top of the vaginal canal. It produces cervical fluid that changes with the menstrual cycle and can be felt at the back of the vagina. During arousal and childbirth, it softens and moves, allowing for both pleasure and the passage of life.

One of my favorite books for really learning about women's genitals and arousal is Sheri Winston's *Women's Anatomy of Arousal*, which goes into great detail and includes many exercises and tips that you will find helpful.

Together, all of these genital parts (including the nipples) form an extensive network of nerve endings. The clitoris alone has over twelve thousand nerve endings, compared to a mere three to four thousand in the penis. Beyond the clitoris, there are significant nerve endings in the perineal and urethral sponges, nipples, inner labia, and the cervix. All of these nerve endings and parts work together to create what Winston calls the *female arousal network*.

So how do you access this network of pleasure? First rule of thumb: Start slowly, and remember that women's arousal is like a cake, not microwave popcorn. Just like the rest of a woman's body, the genitals also need to be warmed up from the outside in. This is especially true for the very sensitive clitoris.

See the Resources section at the end of the book for information about OMG Yes, an app I recommend that provides an in-depth tutorial on how to touch the clitoris and begin learning in the safety and privacy of your own space.

## The G- spot Controversy

When I started my training fifteen years ago, we were taught that the urethral sponge (or G-spot) was a separate organ responsible for G-spot orgasms and female ejaculation (aka "squirting"). More recently, with additional research and MRI imaging studies, consensus is building that there is no particular spot per se, but rather there is a network called the clitourethrovaginal (CUV) complex, a term that describes the sensitive anterior (front) vaginal wall that interacts with the internal part of the clitoris and Skene's (female prostate) glands, which create female ejaculate.

Whatever you decide to call it, stimulation on and around the urethral sponge creates an intense amount of sensation and leads many women to experience a different type of orgasm, which is more intense and can be replicated continuously. It will often include ejaculation because the Skene's glands fill up the urethral sponge with a fluid that is different from urine, although there is usually some urine that does mix with the ejaculate as the fluid comes out through the urethra.

## Learn How to Give a Vulva and Cock Massage

I strongly believe that a picture is worth a thousand words and that when it comes to sex, hands-on learning is the most effective method. It was my heartfelt desire to provide you with videos of what vulva and cock massages look like, but unfortunately, given the climate these days, my legal team nixed it. However, if clients request this and there is full consent, I will walk partners through the process at my private retreats. We also frequently do a sensual massage demonstration at the group retreats as well.

## The Ins and Outs of Female Orgasm

Chapter 13 of my first book, *Living an Orgasmic Life*, provides an in-depth understanding of female orgasm as well as the different types of orgasms that women can experience—clitoral, G-spot, vaginal, and cervical. It also contains many different self-pleasuring rituals which I believe all women, regardless of relationship status, should engage in on a regular basis.

Did you know that for women, orgasm occurs at the intersection of high arousal and high relaxation? In the simplest sense: Orgasm is a release of energy, specifically, of sexual energy. What happens when a body is in contraction? Energy gets stuck and cannot be released. The orgasmic release happens as a result of expanding and opening the body.

Ladies, does this feel familiar? You're fairly high on the arousal scale and feeling close to orgasm. The tension is building, and you start clenching your butt and legs. At the same time, you start holding your breath. But nothing happens. The release doesn't come, and you're left with the female equivalent of "blue balls."

There is a simple reason the orgasm didn't happen: Contracting the body and holding one's breath traps the sexual energy in your genitals, and then it can't be released. The energy literally has no place to go. The remedy for this is to allow breath, sound, and movement to move through your body as your arousal builds.

Breath, sound, and movement are the fuel that feeds the fire of your sexual energy and moves it around your body. My workshops guide women through practices designed to harness and circulate sexual energy throughout the body. As this energy flows, participants often report a cascade effect: first tingling sensations that intensify, then waves of arousal that generate even more energy. I teach specific techniques—deep belly breathing, conscious relaxation and contraction of pelvic floor muscles, fluid hip movements, and sounding—that create pathways for this energy. When done correctly, women describe feeling their arousal continue to build towards orgasm.

## MALE ANATOMY

Male genitalia's external parts (remember: same parts, arranged differently) consist of the penis, foreskin (if uncircumcised), and testicles.

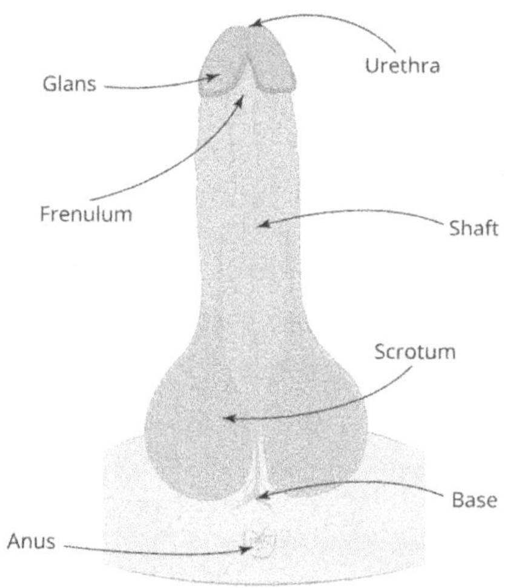


**1. Penis**

- **Root:** It is located underneath the scrotum; the internal base is attached to the pelvic bones, stretching all the way down to the perineum, and contains erectile tissue.
- **Shaft:** The length of the external penis contains erectile tissue.
- **Glans:** The sensitive head or tip, often referred to as the penis head, which is rich in nerve endings (around 3,000–

4,000), making it highly responsive to touch and stimulation. Below the glans is the **penile frenulum**, a thin, highly sensitive fold of tissue that connects the foreskin to the underside of the glans.

**2. Foreskin**

The foreskin is a retractable fold of skin that covers the glans in uncircumcised men. It contains specialized nerve endings that contribute to sexual sensation, which is one of the reasons that men who are uncircumcised tend to have much more sensitivity on their penis.

**3. Scrotum**

The scrotum is the sac of skin that holds the **testicles** outside the body. It contains smooth muscle that contracts or relaxes to raise or lower the testicles in response to temperature or arousal. While there is no erectile tissue in the scrotum, there are many nerve endings, so touching the scrotum can create a lot of pleasurable sensations.

### Internal Genitalia

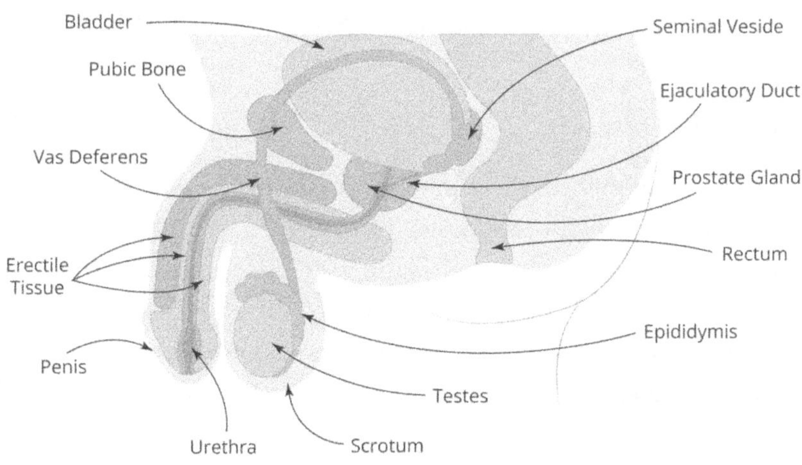

### 1. Testicles (Testes)

The testicles are oval-shaped glands that produce **sperm** and **testosterone**. They're highly sensitive and are a key part of male reproductive and hormonal function.

### 2. Epididymis

A coiled tube located at the back of each testicle, where sperm mature and are stored before ejaculation.

### 3. Vas Deferens

The ducts that transport sperm from the epididymis to the urethra during ejaculation.

### 4. Seminal Vesicles & Prostate Gland

These glands produce the fluid that mixes with sperm to form **semen**. The **prostate** also helps propel semen during ejaculation and contributes to the sensation of orgasm. It's highly sensitive and can be a source of pleasure through internal stimulation.

### 5. Urethra

A tube that runs through the penis, carrying **urine** from the bladder and **semen** from the reproductive system—though not at the same time.

## Male Genital Massage

If you ask men (when their partner is not in the room) how they would rate the touch they receive from their partner, you would be shocked at how low that score might be. This is not to say that most men don't enjoy their partner's touch, but there's a distinction between enjoying touch and receiving an amazing and titillating genital massage, whether by hand or mouth. The truth is that just as most women don't like the way their pussy is touched, many men also would like a different type of touch than what they receive.

However, since penises get aroused much more easily, a man can often still have an orgasm even with mediocre touch.

Here are a few pointers so you can up your game:

- Do not ignore the root or base (internal portion) of the penis. Remember, this is all erectile tissue, just like the shaft, and running your fingers or palm up and down that area can be extremely arousing. If you watch your partner masturbate, which I highly recommend, besides stimulating the shaft, you will likely also see them touching underneath their scrotum, which is where you will find the base.
- Tease the cock (this is also called “edging”). I know you haven’t been taught this, but most men really enjoy having their cock teased (in the right way). Rather than going full throttle, start slower with your hand or tongue. Explore all the different ways you’ve learned to approach touch (Earth, Air, Water, Fire). First, build up arousal in your partner, and then bring them back down by releasing the penis and touching their chest, legs, and belly. Keep on doing this until they are close to orgasm.
- Find their most sensitive spot. Every man knows that there is a place on their penis or a particular type of rhythm or touch that will bring them to orgasm. Find out from your partner where that place is; again, watching them masturbate will give you some good information, and learn the technique.

A book that I highly recommend if you want to learn how to pleasure a penis is Ian Kerner’s book *Passionista: The Empowered Woman’s Guide to Pleasuring a Man.*

## Anal Play

Finally, let's talk about your often-neglected, frequently shamed anus, which can give you immense pleasure. I know that many people shy away from anal play because it feels dirty and embarrassing and we believe anal penetration will hurt. I've learned a lot about anal penetration in the last few years, and I definitely want to encourage you to explore this, both as a giver and a receiver. For many men, anal penetration, whether with a finger or toy, is extremely pleasurable and can significantly enhance their orgasmic potential and experience. The stigma around male penetration has lessened considerably in the last decade as strap-ons have become one of the best sellers in the sexual wellness market.

I still do not hold myself out as the queen of anal play, but I do want you to know the truth versus fiction.

**Some Facts about Anal Play:**

- Your anus has thousands of nerve endings with immense pleasure potential.
- Many nerve endings are right around your butthole. Gently running a finger around the opening can feel amazing. After this experience, you can assess whether you want to explore further.
- Poop is not usually a problem since stool is not stored in the rectum; it's stored deeper in the digestive tract. You can always use latex gloves or do a gentle saline enema beforehand.
- Your G-spot (women) and prostate response (men) can be activated through anal play. Anal stimulation is great for men since it massages the prostate gland, sometimes called the "P-spot." This can help with pelvic pain and prostatitis, improve ejaculatory function, and increase arousal and full

body orgasms. Anal stimulation can also be therapeutic for women with tight pelvic floors. Stimulation can come from fingers, a toy, or a cock; if using a toy, make sure it has a wide base.

- Using lots of lubrication and going very slowly with just one finger is the best way to start. Consider wearing a glove, especially if fingernails have not been trimmed all the way down and thoroughly buffed.
- The more relaxed you are, the more enjoyable the experience, and this is especially true for your butt. Deep breathing into your pelvis is quite helpful.
- Penetrative anal orgasms for women can be mind-blowing, especially if combined with a vaginal orgasm, because the pelvic and pudendal nerves are both involved.
- You can use butt plugs, which can be found in all different sizes, to help open up the anus. I often recommend this for my vaginismus clients and for women and men who are experimenting with anal play for the first time.

If you're interested in exploring anal play further, I highly recommend you read *The Ultimate Guide to Prostate Pleasure* by Charlie Glickman.

We've just reimagined sex—not as a performance, but as an unfolding experience rooted in presence, pleasure, and connection. It's not about doing more, trying harder, or hitting the "right" moves. It's about slowing down, tuning in, and redefining what sex actually means for *you*.

In the next chapter, you'll start to uncover your unique sexual style—the way your body responds, what turns you on, how you like to connect, and how that might differ from your partner. This isn't a one-size-fits-all model. The goal is understanding your own wiring so that intimacy feels natural, nourishing, and sustainable.

# 10

# LEARN YOUR SEXUAL STYLES

Most of us were never taught that we each have a unique erotic blueprint—a specific way our bodies and minds respond to arousal, turn-on, and pleasure. Instead, we learned a one-size-fits-all script for sex, and when that script stopped working, we often assumed something was wrong with us or our relationship.

Nothing could be further from the truth. Just as we have different love languages, we also have different sexual styles or blueprints—patterns of arousal and pleasure that, when understood, can open the door to more connection, more creativity, and a lot more fun in the bedroom.

In this chapter, we'll explore how to identify your own erotic style, understand your partner's, and start speaking each other's pleasure language fluently—so you can stop guessing and start playing in ways that truly light you both up.

There are several different ways to assess your sexual styles; for the purposes of providing you with as complete an understanding as possible, we're going to dive into a few of them.

Sexual styles were first articulated by the psychologist Donald Mosher and popularized by David Schnarch in his best-selling 1997 book *Passionate Marriage: Keeping Love and Intimacy Alive in Committed Relationships*. According to Schnarch, there are three types of sexual styles:

Trance State

Partner Engagement

Role Play and Fantasy

**Trance State**: If you are someone who likes to close your eyes, focus inwardly, and really focus on physical sensation, you are a "trancer." You are likely very kinesthetic, meaning that touch is the primary way you connect with a partner during lovemaking. Trancers tend to like very slow, focused touch. You need minimal distractions; even the slightest interruption can short-circuit your arousal. You can go very deep and even have an out-of-body experience during sex. Emotional connection may be more difficult to maintain because your focus is on your own pleasure rather than on your partner.

**Partner Engagement:** If sex is about emotion, romance, and lots of kissing and eye contact, your sexual style is partner engagement. Intimacy and connection is most important for this style. You like to be romanced with tender, loving words. You need to be in the right mood and prefer a pleasing atmosphere. Partner engagers tend to shy away from casual sexual encounters.

**Role Play and Fantasy**: If you are someone who needs to go into a fantasy in order to get really aroused during sex, or if sex for you is about role play, then this is your sexual style. This style involves a lot of creativity and exploration and the ability and breadth to play many different roles. Role playing requires a fair degree of comfort with your own individuality and sexual expression.

Schnarch's explanation of sexual styles is helpful to an extent but leaves open many questions. How does this relate to someone who likes bondage or Tantra, and what about the person who is genitally focused; where do their styles fit in?

## LEARN YOUR EROTIC BLUEPRINT

Enter Jaiya, an award winning somatic sexologist and sexological body worker colleague. Jaiya is the creator of the Erotic Blueprints Framework™—a system that emerged organically in 2000 following decades of hands-on work. She draws from over thirty years of somatic sexology, during which she worked closely with clients, observing their patterns of arousal, response, and what truly turns them on across physical, psychological, emotional, and spiritual dimensions. Her reach received a tremendous boost in 2021 with the release of the Netflix hit show *Sex, Love and Goop*, in which she was prominently featured, and the subsequent release of her 2023 book *Your Blueprint for Pleasure.*

Jaiya's work is revolutionary, providing people with the vocabulary to comprehend their distinct sexual preferences. It also recognizes that most people don't have just one type of sexual blueprint. Like love languages, we have a primary erotic blueprint, with secondary influences that create our individual erotic blueprint.

The following is used with permission from Jaiya and the Erotic Blueprint Breakthrough™ Program

Jaiya identified five distinct erotic blueprints: Sensual, Energetic, Sexual, Kinky, and Shapeshifter. She also believes that each of these blueprints have a "superpower" as well as a "shadow side," and that it is often the shadow side which creates tension in sexual relationships.

To figure out your erotic blueprint, I highly recommend that you take the Erotic Blueprint Quiz (available at an affordable price), which provides you with an in-depth analysis of your blueprint and how it relates to other blueprints, as well as pleasure practices that you can use immediately. If you really want to take a deep dive into blueprints, join Jaiya's online program, the Erotic Blueprint Breakthrough, which includes hundreds of videos as well as live group coaching with some of her trained coaches.

Let's examine each of the blueprints more closely, and then we will drop into some of my retreat sessions for examples of how you might incorporate your individual blueprints into your sex life.

## Energetic

The Energetic blueprint is all about anticipation, tease, and the invisible field of energy that exists between bodies. People with this blueprint are highly sensitive to subtlety—eye contact, hovering air touch, or even the space between two bodies can be electrifying. Less is more here. They can be turned on by breath, air touch, presence, and spiritual connection, and often need slowness and stillness to fully open up. Individuals who have the energetic blueprint are often drawn to Tantra and sacred sexuality, as well as spiritual practices. For them, sex is a melding of the physical, energetic, emotional and spiritual bodies.

Some of their superpowers are:

- Ability to have energetic, full body, non-ejaculatory (for men) multiple orgasms
- Can sometimes orgasm without being touched
- Can experience altered states of consciousness during orgasm (leave their body, see colors, hear sounds)
- Have a "Spidey sense" that tends to make them very intuitive lovers
- Tend to be empaths and very sensitive to other's emotions and sensations.

But their superpower is also their shadow—too much intensity or too fast a pace can overwhelm their nervous system and shut everything down. Since they are so sensitive to energy, they can easily get bombarded with too many stimuli or other people's energy, which will shut them down. They also may have a harder time staying present during sex due to disassociation or leaving their body.

Energetic sex is so intense and powerful that they might have a hard time enjoying other experiences. There's a saying in the Tantra world, "Once you've experienced Tantric sex, there's no going back." This may be true for some, but there are plenty of other people, myself included, who can easily shift between the energetic and other blueprints.

## Sensual

For the Sensual Blueprint, pleasure is a full-body, multisensory experience. Think candlelight, soft music, luscious fabrics, essential oils, slow melting, earth touch and water touch. A Sensual needs time to warm up—for them foreplay is everything. When all five of their senses are nurtured, they can be wildly orgasmic. The Sensual Blueprint partner thrives on beauty, rhythm, and emotional connection.

These are some of their superpowers:

- They can really drop into their body and experience deep pleasure and sensations (often with their eyes closed, as in a trance state).
- An amazing capacity for pleasure and multisensory orgasms.
- When totally relaxed, they can stay in a highly aroused state for long periods of time without any focus on goals.
- Enjoyment of sensation play; in other words, being touched by objects that create a variety of feelings on the surface of their body, such as feathers or soft plush, sharp objects, or

hot sensations (warm oil, hot paraffin wax) and cold sensations (ice cubes).

The shadow side of the Sensual Blueprint is that they often struggle with getting out of their head and into their body. Their sensual sensitivity can also be a deterrent. They can become easily distracted and disconnect from their body and their pleasure if everything is not perfect (say if the room is too cold or hot, the sheets are itchy, or the music is wrong). They often don't like messes, so they may have an aversion to bodily fluids. Orgasms may also sometimes be elusive —almost there and then gone again.

## SEXUAL

The Sexual Blueprint is what most of us were taught sex is supposed to be: straightforward, genital and orgasm focused, and animalistic, with fire touch. These folks are turned on by nudity, genital stimulation, penetration, and the simplicity of physical turn-on. For them, sex is life-affirming and grounding—and they often feel most emotionally connected through physical connection.

Some of their superpowers are:

- The ability to get turned on very easily and quickly go from zero to sixty
- Often very stimulated by visuals (nudity or porn)
- Very unabashed and can truly embrace pleasure
- Enjoy getting to orgasm and the climax of sexual play
- Can frequently use sex to relax and release tension

The shadow side of the Sexual Blueprint reveals itself when these individuals, accustomed to their own quick-igniting desire, grow impatient with partners who require extended foreplay or emotional connection before becoming aroused.

Since they are frequently so genitally focused, they may miss all the other parts of the body that can experience pleasure. Their goal orientation mindset, aimed at orgasm and penetration, can cause them to miss the whole experience of the journey.

Their challenge is to slow down and explore the richness that exists beyond just "getting to the orgasm."

## KINKY

Kink is often misunderstood, but the Kinky Blueprint isn't just about whips and chains, as unflatteringly portrayed in *Fifty Shades of Grey*. It's about accessing turn-on through taboo—whether that's psychological kink (including dominance/submission and other power exchange play, as well as all kinds of role-playing) or physical kink (restraints, impact play, sensation play). Kinky folks are turned on by the forbidden; they are aroused by breaking the rules in a consensual container. Their eroticism often lives in the realm of creativity and trust. The Kinky Blueprint is perhaps the most expansive of all the blueprints since Kinky play encompasses such a wide variety of sexual play, fantasies, and fetishes. I often describe kink as anything that's not traditional vanilla sex and that in some way pushes societal boundaries of acceptable types of sexual exploration.

Some of their superpowers are:

- Turn-ons, pleasure and orgasms can happen from just playing in the mind
- In deep states of surrender, you can access altered states of consciousness
- May experience deep pleasure from intense sensation or pain
- Can access peak erotic states without penetrative sex
- Can be a very healing experience

The shadow aspects of the Kinky Blueprint often stem from societal judgment and internalized shame. Many kinky individuals feel compelled to conceal their authentic desires due to fear of rejection or stigmatization. Another challenge can be developing dependency on specific scenarios or stimuli for arousal, potentially limiting their pleasure pathways. Additionally, the intense emotional and physical experiences of kinky encounters may lead to what's known as "sub drop" or "dom drop"—a period of post-play emotional or energetic depletion—making proper aftercare an essential component of responsible kinky practice.

## SHAPESHIFTER

As the name implies, the Shapeshifter is the erotic chameleon—the most erotically sophisticated of all the blueprints. They enjoy all the previous blueprints and can easily move from one to the other. They crave variety and novelty, are often highly orgasmic, and are insatiably curious.

The Shapeshifter's superpowers relate to their flexible ability to go in any direction. This makes them versatile and sought-after lovers because they equally enjoy myriad types of erotic and sexual play. Shapeshifters have enormous potential for pleasure and can engage in sexual play for hours at a time. They are never boring and bring an immense depth of creativity and playfulness into relationships.

The shadow side of Shapeshifters is that their adaptability can also be a result of people-pleasing behavior, which may result in them not getting their erotic needs met. Their boundless appetite for diverse experiences can give the impression that they are insatiable, which may be overwhelming to partners. When paired with someone who thrives primarily in just one blueprint, Shapeshifters might find themselves restless, their wandering erotic imagination quietly seeking new horizons beyond what their current relationship offers.

What makes Jaiya's model as set out in the Erotic Blueprint Quiz particularly valuable is how it maps your sexual nature across multiple dimensions. Rather than simply labeling you as one type, it creates a nuanced profile—readily visualized as a pie chart—showing exactly how your desires blend across all five blueprints.

It is extremely rare for an individual to score 100 percent on any one blueprint, and most individuals will notice that they have a variety of erotic languages accessible to them.

A caveat that I always point out to my clients is that the test results are only as accurate as the answers you supply. You also don't know what you don't know and haven't yet experienced. Many of my clients who end up scoring low on one of the blueprints are pleasantly surprised when during a retreat they have the opportunity to explore a new erotic style and learn that it's actually very enjoyable for them. This is particularly true for the sexual styles that are often least familiar: Energetic and Kinky.

I also want to make it abundantly clear that I am not a certified Erotic Blueprint Coach™ and I am not familiar with the details of all the methods that Jaiya teaches in the program to her coaches. However, as a certified Somatica™ sex and intimacy coach and Tantra teacher for over fifteen years, I am very experienced with helping my clients explore many different sexual styles and diverse modes of erotic play that I have learned both through personal experience as well as the extensive number of training programs and workshops I've attended and certifications I've accumulated over the years. I use the Erotic Blueprint to help my clients identify their sexual styles and provide them with a language around erotic play that they can understand and can then explore within the individualized retreat experience I curate for them.

### *Erotic Blueprint Exercise for Couples*

After taking the Erotic Blueprint Quiz and receiving your results, write down the answers to the questions below. Then take a few moments to share and discuss your answers with your partner.

1. What was your primary blueprint, and does it make sense to you? Which of the superpowers can you relate to? Which of the shadow sides of your primary blueprint can you relate to most?
2. Did any of your results for the rest of the blueprints surprise you? Which of them are you most curious about exploring?
3. Comparing your results with your partner's results, how aligned are they? Do the results in any way mirror your experience during sex? Can you identify any patterns from looking at the comparison?

## INTEGRATING YOUR SEXUAL STYLES

**Case Study: Andrea and Kevin**

Meet my clients Andrea and Kevin, who like many of my retreat couples, are struggling with connecting sexually.

"We're never on the same wavelength," Andrea complained. "I want Kevin to slow down, but he's always racing for the finish line."

Kevin shifted uncomfortably in his chair. "I don't understand what takes her so long. By the time she's ready, I've already lost interest. It feels like we're speaking different languages."

They were—literally. When Andrea and Kevin took the Erotic Blueprint Quiz, their results painted a clear picture of the sexual disconnection they were experiencing with each other. Andrea scored highest as a Sensual (45 percent) with secondary Energetic influences (25 percent), while Kevin was predominantly Sexual (55 percent) with some Kinky leanings (20 percent).

"This explains everything," Andrea said, studying her results. As a Sensual, she needed the full sensory experience—dimmed lights, luxurious textures, and extended foreplay that engaged all her senses. Kevin's erotic blueprint meant he was aroused quickly by direct genital touch and visual stimulation—and was ready to move toward orgasm within minutes of physical contact.

"So I'm not broken?" Kevin asked, looking genuinely relieved. "And she's not just trying to slow things down to frustrate me?"

"Not at all," I explained. "You're both perfectly normal, just wired differently. Think of it like this: Andrea needs to simmer before she boils, while you, Kevin, go from cold to boiling almost instantly."

During our first session, I had them create a sensory experience together. I guided Kevin in slowing down and engaging Andrea's senses one by one—lighting candles, playing soft music, using scented massage oil to touch her with sensuous water and air touch.

"This feels...different," Kevin admitted afterward. "I was actually getting turned on by how turned on she was becoming."

Andrea smiled. "And I was really able to relax, because I wasn't worried about having to perform. Kevin's touch felt so good, and he actually seemed present and focused on me the whole time."

"Let's try deepening Andrea's sensual experience," I suggested, while bringing out the sensual tool kit that I offer to all my clients.

"Ooh, this looks like fun!" Kevin exclaimed with a glint in his eye.

My sensual tool kit consists of different sensory objects ranging from soft objects like feathers, silk scarves, and a fuzzy massage mitt to sharper objects—a 'vampire' mitt, a small metal flogger that's great for hot and cold sensation play, and a small nickel sized wheel with sharp spikes you can carefully run over the skin (aka a Wartenberg wheel).

During our sensation play session, Andrea learned that she loved to begin with light, feathery touch, but as she became more aroused, she started enjoying some more intense sensations. The vampire mitt (a big furry mitt with tacks on one side) was one of her favorites, especially when Kevin brushed it very lightly on her back.

"This is really turning me on," Kevin said, "seeing how much Andrea is enjoying all these sensations."

I laughed, "I'm not surprised, and you'll be thrilled to know that sensation play is in the realm of the kink world."

Kevin's eyes widened. "Really? This counts as kinky?"

"Absolutely," I confirmed. "Kink isn't just about leather and dungeons. It's about exploring sensations and power dynamics that exist outside conventional sexual scripts. Sensation play is absolutely within that realm, and it's a wonderful bridge between Andrea's Sensual Blueprint and your Kinky tendencies."

**Building Your Sensual Toolkit**

If you come to my Passion in Paradise Group Retreat, you will be directed to build and bring your own sensual tool kit (because I have limits on how much luggage I can manage internationally!) Anyone can build their own sensual tool kit, and you don't have to break the bank to do it. Start looking around your home, check your kitchen or closet, and I guarantee you will find many sensual objects you can add to that kit. Here are some ideas:

- Feather duster
- Silk robe tie or silk tie
- Scarf
- Furry stuffed animal

- Avocado oil (one of my faves)
- Fork (sharper sensations)
- Heavy metal chain
- Essential oils and/or a diffuser
- Chocolate, fresh strawberries, and/or whipped cream
- Small brush or toothbrush
- Metal head scratcher

If you want a "Made for You" sensation play kit, check out the store on my website at: www.passionateintimacyretreats.com/store

**Back to Kevin and Andrea:**

"It's important that we also honor Kevin's Sexual Blueprint," I told them both. "Andrea, I want you to understand that Kevin's direct approach isn't about him being selfish, but is simply his natural arousal pattern."

Andrea nodded thoughtfully. "I think I could do that. It's just that when I close my eyes, I go so deep into the sensations."

"You don't have to keep them open the whole time," I clarified. "Think of it as making periodic check-ins—a moment of eye contact, a deliberate touch, and then you can return to your internal focus. Kevin, this means you'll need to be patient for those longer stretches when Andrea is in her sensual trance."

"I can work on that," Kevin said, though I could hear the uncertainty in his voice. "But what if I lose my arousal waiting?"

"That's a great question," I told him. "Let's be clear, though, that there's a difference between losing your erection and losing your arousal. It's normal for a man's erection to come and go during foreplay, especially if a lot of your attention is directed towards Andrea."

"I'm always concerned that if I lose it, I won't get it back," Kevin told us both.

"That's typically not the case," I reassured him. "Both men's erections and women and men's arousal can rise and fall, but they will come back once there's more physical stimulation. Andrea, one way you can help Kevin is to every so often touch his penis during the initial phase of foreplay to keep him engaged. You can also give him other cues like making sounds, telling him it feels good, and directing him to touch you in a way you would like to be touched."

When Andrea and Kevin came to our next session, they reported that they had been exploring each other's sexual styles at home.

"We created a ritual," Andrea explained with newfound enthusiasm. "We start with what we call 'blueprint trading'—fifteen minutes focused on my sensual needs, then fifteen on Kevin's sexual needs."

Kevin nodded eagerly. "It's been eye-opening. I never realized how much anticipation could enhance my experience. When I slow down and focused on Andrea's pleasure, I actually stayed more aroused than usual. It was like her enjoyment fed mine."

This is a common discovery for couples who begin speaking each other's erotic language. The blueprint framework isn't about compromise—it's about expansion. By understanding and occasionally stepping into the realm of your partner's primary erotic language, you can develop new neural pathways for pleasure that might have otherwise remained dormant.

## SEXUAL PRACTICE: EDGING

For those with a primary Sexual Blueprint, the practice of edging can be very erotic. It also is very helpful for men who have challenges with early ejaculation. Edging means that you bring your partner (or yourself) up and down on the arousal scale through direct genital stimulation.

For men, edging involves direct stimulation until he approaches climax—around a seven or eight on a ten-point arousal scale—then pausing just before the point of no return. During this pause, redirect sensation by touching other parts of his body—arms, chest, neck, legs, and so on—allowing arousal to subside slightly before beginning the cycle again. This rhythmic approach-and-retreat pattern builds intensity while extending pleasure.

For men with ejaculation issues who often have difficulty distinguishing between different levels of arousal, this practice will help them to learn what the various arousal levels feel like. The aim is for them to develop the ability to sustain increasingly higher arousal levels for extended durations.

For women, the process is similar but will involve directly touching her clitoris or G-spot, moving her slowly towards and away from orgasm. This type of extended teasing can produce incredibly intense orgasms when she's finally allowed to climax. Some women discover they can experience multiple peaks this way, with each successive wave becoming more powerful than the last.

## PLAYING WITH ENERGY

In our next session, I introduced Andrea and Kevin to Energetic Blueprint practices that would complement Andrea's secondary erotic language while offering Kevin a completely new experience.

"Today we're going to explore energetic touch and play, which form the foundation of sacred sexuality and Tantra," I explained. "The Cliff Notes version of Energetics is to understand that we are all just made up of atoms of energy, both inside and outside of our body. In the world of Tantra, we have seven energy centers inside our body called chakras, which you may have heard of from your yoga practice, Andrea."

"Yes," she replied. "Our teacher often refers to our root chakra when we do a grounding exercise at the end of class."

"Precisely," I continued. "You can think of these chakras as wheels that spin in a circle. They also can be open or closed, like petals on a flower. The chakras are lined up vertically, stretching from the base of your perineum to the top of your head; imagine them stacked up in a hollow tube."

I pointed to the chakra ladder hanging in my office. "Each chakra represents a different element: earth, water, fire, air, sound, light, and thought. They are also connected to different colors and sounds, as well as emotions.

CHAKRA COLORS & MEANINGS
CROWN
Sahasara
Violet
Top of the Head
Thought
▸ Enlightenment & Spirituality Consciousness
Excessive: Overly Intellectual, Confusion, Spiritual Addiction, Dissociation
Deficient: Limited Beliefs, Apathy
Balanced: Wisdom, Knowledge, Spiritual Connection, Consciousness
THIRD EYE
Ajna, Indigo
Above / Between Eyebrows
Light
▸ Intuition & Understanding
Excessive: Headaches, Nighmares, Delusions, Difficulty, Concentrating
Deficient: Poor Memory, Poor Vision, Unimaginitive, Dental
Balanced: Psychic Perception, Accurate Interpretation, Imagination, Clear Seeing
THROAT
Vishuddha
Blue
Center base of Neck
Sound
▸ Comminucation & Self - Expression
Excessive: Inability to Listen, Stuttering Excessive Talking
Deficient: Fear of Speaking, Poor Rythm
Balanced: Clear Communication, Creativity, Resonance
HEART
Anahata
Green
Center of Chest
Air
▸ Balance, Love & Connection
Excessive: Codependency, Jealous, Possessive, Poor Boundaries
Deficient: Shy, Lonely, Isolated, Bitter
Balanced: Compassion, Balance, Self Acceptance, Good Relationships
SOLAR PLEXUS
Manipura
Yellow
Below Sternum
Fire
▸ Energy, Vitality, Will Power, Desire, Personal Authority
Excessive: Dominating, Controlling, Aggressive, Scattered
Deficient: Poor Self Esteem, Passive
Balanced: Vitality, Strength of Will, Purpose, Self Esteem
SACRAL
Svadhisthana
Orange
Below Navel
Water
▸ Relationship, Emotions & Sexuality, Self Gratification
Excessive: Overly Emotional, Sex Addiction, Obsessive Attachments
Deficient: Rigid, Emotionally Numb
Balanced: Healthy Sexually, Pleasure, Feeling, Fluidity
ROOT
Muladhara
Red
Base of Spine
Earth
▸ To Be Here, Grounded, Survival, Self Preservation
Excessive: Obesity, Greed, Materialism, Hoarding, Sluggish
Deficient: Fearful, Underweight, Spacey
Balanced: Stability, Grounded, Prosperity, Physically Healthy, Trust

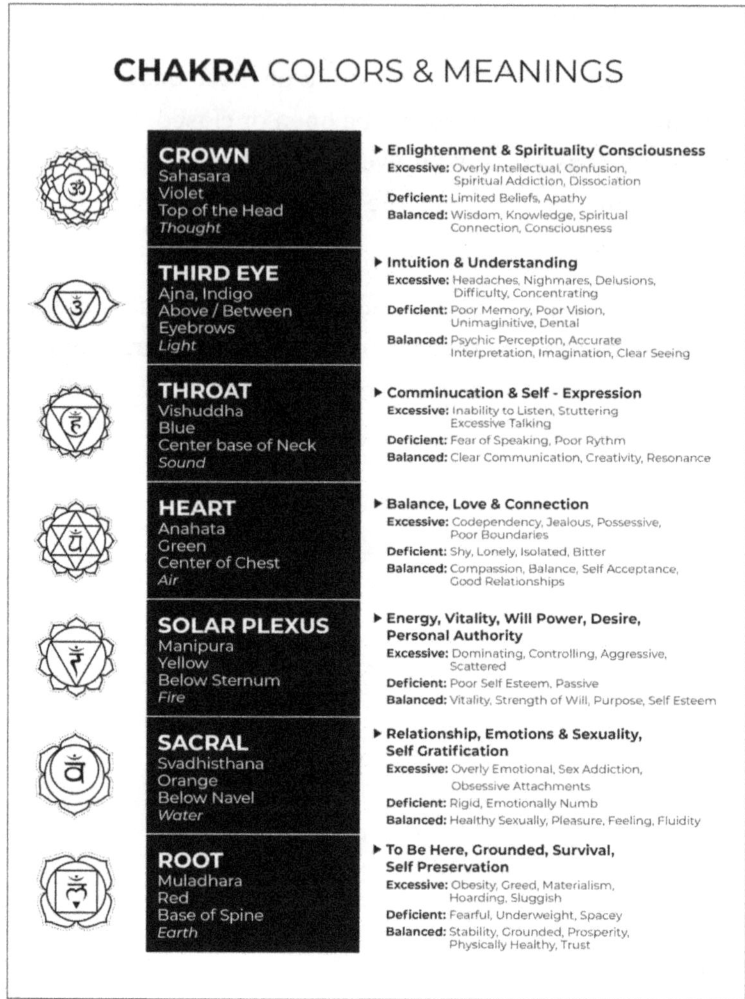

"The important piece to understand about chakras is that when properly activated through breath, sound, movement, and touch, they help us activate our sexual energy and move it through our body to reach orgasmic states."

"This sounds pretty woo-woo to me," Kevin demurred, with skepticism in his voice.

"I totally understand that," I replied. "But honestly, these chakras have always been present in our vernacular. You've heard stingy people being called 'tight-assed,'" at which they both laughed. "Well, our first chakra is all about survival, so in Tantra, a stingy person would be seen as having a deficient first chakra." Kevin nodded.

"I bet you've also heard the saying "he has fire in his belly" for someone who is assertive and ambitious?"

"That would be my boss," Kevin wryly commented.

I continued, "Our third chakra is our power center—-when it's properly activated, you feel powerful. When it's deficient, you may feel anxious and have 'butterflies in your stomach.'"

"What about having a 'broken heart'?" Andrea asked.

"Exactly," I agreed with a smile. "That's your heart chakra, the fourth energy center. When it's open, you feel loving, compassionate, and connected. When it's wounded or closed, you might feel grief, especially around being abandoned, or have difficulty giving and receiving love."

I guided them through a simple exercise to feel energy between their palms. "Place your hands together, palm to palm. Close your eyes and rub your palms together until you feel a bit of warmth between them. Now separate your hands about eight inches apart and imagine you are holding a Nerf football between your two palms. Place all of your intention on the football between your two hands. Now slowly move your hands slightly closer, then farther apart."

Kevin's eyebrows shot up. "I actually feel something—like a magnetic resistance!" he exclaimed.

"That's energy," I confirmed. "Now imagine sending that energy to Andrea without touching her."

I had them sit face-to-face, eyes closed, palms hovering inches from each other's bodies.

"This is weird," Kevin stated at first, but then he was surprised to find the process aroused him too. "I can actually feel something between my hand and her skin—like heat or electricity."

Andrea's eyes were closed, her breath deepening. "It's like electricity," she whispered. "Keep going."

As it became clear they were both able to access energy, I showed Kevin how he could play with Andrea's energy by putting more attention and intention into his hands, since energy follows intention.

"My hands just got warmer," he declared with surprise in his voice. Andrea's body immediately responded with some minor quivering, and she also told us she was seeing an orange color. Kevin looked up at me with some alarm.

"This is totally normal," I told them. "When energy moves through your body, it can manifest itself in different ways. It's not uncommon for you to feel warmth or tingling, or even experience involuntary shaking or slight tremors, which we call "krias" in Tantra. They are totally harmless." I could see the relief on Kevin's face.

"It's also indicating that you may have easy access to full body orgasms," I added. "There are also many other ways to access energy, and the visual—seeing colors—is also one of the ways that Andrea experiences energy."

"But why am I seeing orange?" Andrea asked.

"There's no way to know for sure," I explained. "But in Tantra, your second or sacral chakra, which is your sexual center, is depicted as orange, so it's likely that you're experiencing a lot of sexual energy in your body right now."

Andrea laughingly affirmed, "Yes, I'm ready to stop our session and go back to our room, right now!"

For a much more expansive discussion of Tantra, including its origins, as well as much more detailed information about the chakras, I recommend that you read Chapter 10, "So What is Tantra Anyway?" in my book *Living an Orgasmic Life*. I also include many other references if you'd really like to dive deeper into the world of Tantra.

## *COUPLES CHAKRA SOUNDING ENERGY PRACTICE*

A great way to connect with each other's chakras and to start to identify what they feel like when they're activated is to engage in this chakra sounding exercise.

1. Partner One lies down on the bed or floor, closes their eyes, and begins gentle breathing.
2. Partner Two kneels or sits down next to Partner One and gently places their mouth about 3 to 4 inches over Partner One's root chakra, located at their perineum, which is between their legs, right below the genitals, and is known in American slang as the 'taint.' They make the sound *Lamm* three times, focusing on the final sound (*Mmm*), which creates vibration. Partner One just breathes gently and notices what they're feeling in their body.
3. Partner Two then places their mouth 3 to 4 inches over Partner One's genitals at the sacral chakra and makes the sound *Vomm* three times.
4. Partner Two then moves to the solar plexus, located in the center of the recipient's body right below the rib cage (or bra line) and makes the sound *Romm* three times.

5. Partner Two then moves to the heart chakra, located in the center of the chest (not the left side where the anatomical heart lives), and makes the sound *Yomm* three times.
6. At the throat chakra (base of the throat), Partner Two makes the sound *Homm* three times.
7. Now move to their third eye, right in the middle of their forehead, about two inches above the eyebrows, and make the sound *Ohmm* three times. Some caution is advised here since many highly intuitive and energetically sensitive people can experience quite a bit of sensation in this area, I always suggest that you tone the volume of your sound down at this energy center. If your partner reacts or tells you they are experiencing too much intensity, pull your mouth back to six or eight inches away from the third eye.
8. For the crown chakra, which is located at the top of the head, Partner Two places a finger gently in each of Partner One's ears, blocking them up. This chakra sounding is silent, except for any internal sound that Partner One experiences with their ears blocked off (which may include buzzing, pulsing, or other inner sounds).
9. When complete, Partner One then rests for a minute or two, taking some deep breaths, and then slowly starts moving their fingers and toes and gradually opens their eyes.
10. Switch so that Partner Two can receive.
11. At the end of the practice, discuss what it felt like for each of you, both giving and receiving. What sensations did you feel? Was there a particular chakra that felt more alive or more closed? Did you notice anything else (colors, shapes, images, or sounds)?

**Surprise: Andrea is Kinky Too!**

For Andrea and Kevin's final session of the retreat, we explored Kevin's secondary language of kink. Unfortunately, kinky people have often been condemned in society—called out as freaks, mislabeled as pedophiles, or assumed to have trauma or unresolved psychological issues. This stigma keeps many people from exploring their authentic desires, even within committed relationships.

“I want to be clear that kink isn't about violence or disrespect," I explained to both of them. "At its core, kink is about consensual power exchange, heightened sensation, and exploring the psychological aspects of arousal. It requires tremendous trust and communication—often more than conventional sex.”

Andrea looked intrigued but uncertain. “I scored so low on Kinky that I assumed it wasn't for me.”

“Remember what I said about not knowing what you don't know,” I reminded her. “Your Sensual Blueprint actually has a lot of overlap with certain types of kink—especially sensation play, which we've already discovered you enjoy.”

Andrea smiled, acknowledging, “I did love that.”

“And kink exists on a vast spectrum,” I continued. “We're not talking about anything extreme—just some light exploration that might surprise you both."

I started by having them explore power dynamics through simple eye contact, placing them face-to-face at one end of my office with Kevin’s back to the wall.

“Kevin, using your eyes only, I want you to move Andrea to the other side of the room.” Kevin looked up at me quizzically.

Then I demonstrated to Kevin how I could wordlessly give a command simply through my eyes. First, I looked at him sweetly. Then I looked at him like I owned him, sending out the energy of “you’re mine, and you’re going to do what I tell you to do.” Kevin’s whole body immediately shifted, his head lowered a bit, and his shoulders dropped in submission to my command.

“Wow,” Kevin said quietly. “I actually felt that power shift. It was...intense.”

“That’s power exchange in its most subtle form. Now you try it with Andrea,” I instructed.

Kevin's first attempt was hesitant, but after a few tries and a little coaching, his gaze transformed as he locked eyes with Andrea. His eyes darkened, his posture straightened, and a subtle confidence emerged. Without a word, he directed Andrea with just his eyes, gesturing slightly toward the other side of the room.

Andrea hesitated momentarily, then slowly began moving backward as Kevin continued to move with her, leaving a foot and a half between their bodies. Andrea’s breath quickened visibly as she responded to his silent command.

“How did that feel?” I asked when she reached the far wall.

“Unexpectedly...exciting,” she admitted, a flush creeping up her neck. “Like something inside me wanted to both resist and surrender at the same time.”

“That's the dance of dominance and submission,” I explained. “It's about the exchange of power, not force. The submissive actually holds tremendous power in the dynamic because everything happens with their consent.”

Kevin smiled, clearly intrigued by this revelation. “I never thought about it that way—that the submissive partner holds power too.”

“Absolutely,” I affirmed. “In healthy BDSM dynamics, the submissive sets boundaries and can stop everything with a *safe word*. It's actually built on deep trust and communication.”

“Now, let’s switch,” I told them. I was curious to see how Andrea would respond to being in control.

Much to Andrea's surprise, but not mine, she immediately assumed a dominant role, looking down at Kevin with assumed authority. Without any hesitation, she quickly moved Kevin across the room with her eyes.

"How did that feel, Andrea?" I asked. "That was amazing," she said.

Her voice carried a newfound confidence that seemed to surprise even herself. "I felt... powerful. Like I could make him do anything I wanted." She glanced at Kevin with a mischievous smile. "And he looked like he wanted to let me."

Kevin nodded, his cheeks slightly flushed. "I've never experienced anything like that. When Andrea looked at me that way, my whole body just...responded. I wanted to please her."

"This is what I mean about not knowing what you don't know," I reminded them, smiling at Andrea's obvious surprise at her own dominant capacity. "Many people who score low on Kinky simply haven't had the opportunity to explore these dynamics safely."

"I didn't think I would like this," Andrea told me, "But I'm really turned on."

"That's beautiful," I emphasized. "You're both discovering that you can access different aspects of power exchange. Kevin, your primary Sexual Blueprint often correlates with dominant energy, but you clearly enjoy submission too. And Andrea, your sensual nature can absolutely encompass the psychological control aspects of dominance."

For their final kinky exploration, I introduced them to sensation play with temperature. "This combines Andrea's Sensual Blueprint with Kevin's Kinky interests," I explained, bringing out a bowl of ice cubes and a mug of warm massage oil.

I instructed Kevin to place a blindfold on Andrea. "Kevin, I want you to alternate between the ice and warm oil on her arms and shoulders. Don't tell her which one is coming next."

Kevin dipped his fingers in the warm oil first, trailing them slowly down Andrea's arm. She sighed contentedly, melting into the familiar sensual touch. Then, without warning, he pressed an ice cube to the same spot.

Andrea gasped and arched away from the sensation but didn't ask him to stop. "Oh my God," she breathed.

"How does that feel?" I asked.

"Intense. Shocking. But...I want more."

I laughed.

Kevin alternated between the ice and warm oil for several more minutes, with each contrast drawing increasingly vocal responses from Andrea. The unpredictability clearly heightened her arousal—not knowing whether the next touch would be soothing warmth or shocking cold kept her nervous system engaged in a completely new way.

"This is what we call 'sensation play,'" I explained to Kevin as he continued. "The element of surprise, the contrast between sensations, and yes—the slight edge of not knowing what's coming next, that's psychological kink."

When they finished, Andrea pulled off the blindfold, her eyes bright with discovery. "I had no idea my body could respond like that. Not knowing what was coming made everything so much more intense."

"And how was that for you, Kevin?" I asked.

"Incredible," he said immediately. "Watching her reactions, having that control over her pleasure—it was such a turn-on."

This final session had revealed something profound for both of them: Andrea wasn't just tolerating Kevin's kinky interests; she was discovering her own. The blueprint framework had opened a door to mutual exploration rather than compromise.

As we wrapped up their retreat, I asked them to reflect on what they'd learned about themselves and each other.

“I think the biggest revelation for me,” Andrea said thoughtfully, “is that I'm not just one thing. I always thought of myself as this sensual, slow-to-warm-up person who needed candles and romance. But there's this whole other side of me that can be dominant and loves the edge of kink.”

Kevin nodded. “And I've discovered that slowing down doesn't mean losing intensity—sometimes it actually increases it. When I take time to explore Andrea's sensual side, I find new aspects of pleasure I never knew existed. I can’t wait to explore more with Andrea when we get home.”

## End of Chapter Notes:

My intention for this chapter is to introduce you to a range of sexual styles and to let you see how different expressions of sexuality can coexist and complement one another within a relationship. The more expansive forms of sexuality, such as kink and energetics, carry with them their own philosophies, practices, and ethical foundations, including the importance of consent, safety, and self-awareness. Rather than attempting to be exhaustive, this chapter is designed to help you begin to orient yourself within this broader context of sexuality and recognize what resonates for you and your partner. If your interest has been sparked, I encourage you to explore the books and other resources included in the Resources section at the end of this book, which offer a variety of paths to deepening your understanding so that you can continue your learning beyond these pages, as well as offering the opportunity to engage with me more directly.

Now that we've redefined sex as something far richer than just performance or penetration, the next step is getting curious about what truly turns you on—not just physically, but emotionally. Because at its core, desire isn't just about friction and sensation; it's about the feelings we long to experience during sex. Power, surrender, freedom, safety, being wanted, being in control—your unique turn-ons often reveal the deeper emotional truths that live in your body. In the next chapter, we'll explore how fantasies and peak sexual experiences can help you uncover your core desires and create more connected, satisfying, and passionate intimacy.

# 11

# EXPLORING CORE DESIRES AND FANTASIES

To build a lifetime of passionate intimacy, you must first understand the emotional landscape beneath your sexual desires. When asked what they want from sex, most people default to physical sensations: "I want to feel aroused, excited, tingling all over." While these bodily responses matter, they're merely surface expressions of deeper emotional currents—the true place of your desires. Unfortunately, most couples are not aware of this, and so they end up focusing on just the physical aspects of sex, which after a while will become rote and boring, resulting in decreasing desire and lower libido.

Let me give you an example from my own life. As my sexual awakening journey continued to unfold, I was increasingly able to understand my arousal pattern and ask for what I wanted. Sex with various partners felt good, even great sometimes, and I reached higher levels of pleasure and orgasmic bliss. Because much of my awakening happened in the realm of Tantra, where the focus is on worshipping the Goddess, I had several years of beautiful experiences with kindhearted, gentle lovers who put my pleasure first.

Then I met Paul, a six foot three hunk of a man with deep-set eyes who swept me off my feet. Unlike my Tantra lovers, Paul had very strong, masculine, dominant energy. His voice was commanding, both in and out of the bedroom, and our sex was intense and passionate. He slowly introduced me to some light bondage; blindfolds, light restraints, and domination, which my body embraced in a way that no Tantra lover had been able to help me discover. I loved the feeling of losing control and totally surrendering to his power.

I'll never forget my first experience of sub space. It was as if I'd slipped through a crack in reality—time ceased to exist, and my physical body dissolved as waves of pleasure coursed through it and my consciousness floated away from the room. Nothing else—no meditation retreat, no massage, no other intimate encounter—has ever matched the profound surrender and peace I find when I slip into sub space with someone I deeply trust. It is an experience my body craves, and it is the heart of my sexual desires.

While this experience with Paul helped me clarify that I had a kinky side to me and that any future partner would also have to embrace kink, it wasn't until I went through my Somatica training in 2013 that I learned where these desires come from.

## CORE DESIRES

In essence, your core desires are the set of feelings that you want to have during sex which unlocks your arousal. The concept of Core Desires was first conceived by the founders of Somatica, Danielle Harel and Celeste Hirschman, in their 2019 book *Coming Together.* However, it's important to note that Harel and Hirschman built upon the seminal work of the renowned psychotherapist Jack Morin, who wrote *The Erotic Mind: Unlocking the Inner Sources of Passion and Fulfillment* in 1995.

Morin discusses the concept of a “core erotic theme” consisting of the people, images, and experiences that turn you on and are the most arousing for you. He believes that your core erotic theme always has a direct connection with your past challenges and difficulties. In studying the fantasies and peak sexual experiences of thousands of individuals, he found that their sexual desires were related to past childhood experiences and an obstacle that they had to overcome. In his view, the frustration of overcoming these obstacles became our deepest turn-ons or core erotic themes.

Danielle Harel and Celeste Hirschman significantly expanded upon Morin’s work and connected core childhood wounds to the concept of core desires. They discovered that “Erotic desires are a direct attempt to soothe childhood wounds, including everything from our lack of getting a certain set of core needs met to experiences of trauma.” According to the authors, these core desires are an attempt to soothe our childhood wounds, either by Resolution or by Repetition with Agency, which will be described in more detail later in this chapter. Also, because your core desires, just like your core childhood wounds, are immutable, what turns you on will not change over time, although how you get there might.

**Case Study: Tamara and Craig**

Like many couples that I see, Tamara and Craig were struggling with mismatched desires. Craig wanted sex much more frequently than Tamara, who consistently made excuses. After only having had sex twice in the previous six months, Craig was at a breaking point when they attended one of my private retreats.

During our first session together, I could see the tension between them—Craig's frustration manifesting as nervous energy, and Tamara's withdrawal, evident in her crossed arms and minimal eye contact.

“Let's start by understanding what sex means to each of you,” I suggested, creating a safe container for honest conversation. “Beyond the physical sensations, what emotional experiences are you seeking?”

Craig shifted uncomfortably. “I feel like I'm just another task on her to-do list,” Craig confessed, his voice tight with frustration. “I want to be wanted.”

Tamara sighed, twisting her wedding ring. “I'm exhausted all the time. When he touches me, it feels like pressure to be perfect, to respond in certain ways, to make sure Craig's needs are being met. It's exhausting.”

“Tamara,” I gently prodded. “When you do have sex with Craig, how would you describe what sex looks like?”

She gave Craig a sideways glance, and he nodded his head for her to continue. “He's always very sweet with me. It starts with gentle kissing, then he might touch my boobs, go down on me, ask me for a blow job, and then we have sex.”

“That sounds pretty typical,” I told them. “What feelings come up for you during sex?” I pried deeper.

“If I'm being totally honest,” Tamara said sheepishly, “it's really boring for me. Everything's routine, and I never feel any excitement or passion from Craig.”

Craig's face fell, clearly expressing hurt at her admission. “I didn't know you felt that way,” he said quietly. “I've been trying to be gentle and considerate because I thought that's what you wanted.”

I nodded, recognizing a pattern I'd seen countless times before. “This is actually very common. Craig, you've been giving Tamara what you thought she wanted—tenderness and consideration. But Tamara, it sounds like something is missing for you emotionally during these encounters.”

Tamara nodded vigorously, seeming relieved that someone understood. “Yes! I mean, I appreciate that he's sweet, but it feels...I don't know, predictable? Safe? There's no surprise, no intensity.”

“This is a great time to explore both of your core desires, or the feelings that you truly want to have from sex,” I explained.

“Before I guide you through a visualization exercise, let’s talk about how you’re going to identify what those core desires are,” I told them.

“In this exercise, I’m going to ask you to work with one of three different scenarios:

(1) a peak sexual experience that you’ve had with any partner—a time when you were the most excited and aroused.

(2) a common fantasy that you go to when you want to get turned on, often during masturbation.

(3) something that hasn’t happened yet, but if it did happen, it would be an incredible turn-on for you.”

Craig immediately spoke up, “I have a fantasy that I can work with”

“Great; what about you, Tamara? Can you find something here that resonates?”

From the look on Tamara’s face, I could see that she was really struggling. Her brow furrowed, and she stared down at her hands for what felt like several minutes. “I honestly can't think of anything,” she finally whispered. “I don't really have fantasies, and I can't remember a time when sex was...you know, amazing.”

This was not uncommon either. Many women, particularly those in long-term relationships, struggle to connect with their authentic sexual desires, held back by sexual shame and societal conditioning around female masturbation.

I could also feel Craig's energy shift beside her, his body tensing with what I recognized as both hurt and surprise. But I kept my focus on Tamara, maintaining a gentle, nonjudgmental tone.

"That's okay, Tamara. It's more common than you might think. Let's try the third option—something that hasn't happened but would be incredibly arousing if it did. Sometimes our bodies know what we want even when our minds haven't caught up yet. It might be helpful to think about a scene from a favorite book or movie that was a turn-on for you."

She was quiet for a long moment, her fingers working nervously at her wedding ring. I waited, allowing the silence to create space for whatever wanted to emerge.

"There is...something," she finally whispered, still not making eye contact with either one of us. "Go on," I gently encouraged her. "I really loved the book *Fifty Shades of Grey*. There were some scenes in there that really turned me on."

Craig's eyebrows shot up in surprise. "*Fifty Shades*? Seriously?" The disbelief in his voice was palpable.

I nodded encouragingly at Tamara.

"That's excellent, Tamara. Many women connected deeply with that book precisely because it tapped into desires they hadn't fully acknowledged. Can you share what specifically about those scenes resonated with you?"

"I loved the way Christian took complete control and Ana didn't have to think or make any decisions. The scene in the elevator where he was controlling her vibrator through a remote control was so hot," she said a little breathlessly.

"Fantastic, Tamara," I said. "Now you can use some elements from the book to create the experience that you would like to have when we do the visualization exercise."

"I can't wait to hear what you come up with," Craig said with a little excitement in his voice.

### *Core Desire Visualization Exercise*

(A modified version included with permission from Danielle Harel and Celeste Hirschman from their book *Coming Together: Embracing Your Core Desires for Sexual Fulfillment and Long-Term Compatibility.*)

1. Close your eyes and ground yourself. Start noticing your body and how it feels at this moment. Stretch, move, or do anything you need to do to settle into your body.
2. Take a deep breath into your chest; another deep breath into your belly; a third deep breath into your pelvis, and gently squeeze your PC muscle a few times.
3. As you continue to breathe with gentle PC muscle contractions, I invite you to start imagining one of three scenarios: the hottest sexual experience that you have ever had, a fantasy that would most likely make you reach orgasm, or a sexual experience that you would really like to have, but haven't had yet.
4. Once you've landed on the scene that you want to work with, begin to embody it by building the scene with as many details as possible:

- Where are you? (Are you inside in a room or outside in nature?)
- Who is there with you? (Are you alone, or with others?)
- What does the place look like? (What colors do you see? What's above you and below you?)
- What are you sitting on, standing on, or lying down on?.
- What smells do you notice?
- What sensations are you having on your skin? (for example, sweaty, gooseflesh or chill bumps, hot, cold, or prickly?)
- What are you wearing or not wearing?

- What are other people in your scene wearing or not wearing?
- What is happening in the scene? Are these actions happening to you or to others? You can also be observing rather than participating—that's totally fine.
- Let yourself focus on this scene, and zero in on the thing that really turns you on.

5. As you are seeing and experiencing the scene with as many details as possible, start to notice the feeling you really want to have. What really matters to you?

You may feel:
Loved, calm, degraded, powerful, free, precious, beautiful, connected, considered, playful, fun, vulnerable, pushed, open, received, dominant, collaborative, played with, exploitative, manipulative, taken advantage of, used, naughty, afraid, scared, penetrated, approved of, forced, encouraged, adventuresome, ravished, seen, dissolved, shamed, impressive, authentic, consumed, united, generous, spiritual, trusted, punished, out of control, open, accepted, powerful, free, not responsible, transcendent, appreciated, in control, celebrated, capable, sexy, taken, probed, submissive, understood, safe, taboo, valued, adored, secretive, exposed, controlled, feminine, masculine, androgynous, accepted, cruel, teased, irresistible, merged, unattainable, worshipped, contained, pleasing, mysterious, supported.

There may be some other words or feelings or moments that really help you sense what you want to deeply feel when you go to sex...and you may have several conflicting emotions, and that's okay too.

6. Identify the first feeling that comes to you. Let yourself really feel those feelings, let them spread through your body. Go back to your scene and notice what makes you feel like that. Is it the actions, the

environment, the relationship between you and others or between those you are watching or who are watching you? Is it a particular type of person, or object, or certain words or phrases?
7. Repeat this step for as many feelings as you've identified. When complete, take a nice deep breath and come back to the room.
8. Write down the feelings and the scene that you were working with and acknowledge each of the feelings which form your Core Desires.
9. As a partner exercise, I suggest first sharing the feelings that you want to have. You can decide whether it's safe to also share the scene that you are working with. This can be triggering, so be mindful of where your relationship is and how much skill you both have in dealing with uncomfortable conversations and conflict.

Let's listen in to some more of Tamara and Craig's session:

After completing the visualization exercise, I asked them to each share the feelings they had identified.

Craig volunteered to go first. He took a deep breath, his hands clasped tightly in his lap. "The main feeling I identified was...desired. I want to feel wanted and irresistible. In my fantasy, my partner can't keep her hands off me. She initiates, she pursues me, she makes it clear that she needs me." His voice grew quieter. "I also want to feel appreciated—like my touch and my attention are gifts, not obligations."

I nodded, watching Tamara's face carefully as she absorbed this information. Her expression had softened considerably.

"Thank you for sharing that, Craig. Those are beautiful desires. Tamara, are you ready to share?"

She nodded slowly, though I could see her hands trembling slightly. "The strongest feeling was...not being responsible. I want to feel completely taken care of, where I don't have to think or decide anything. Submissive also came up for me."

"Great, Tamara," I said. "Are you open to sharing with Craig the scene that you were working with?" Tamara took a deep breath and then began to share.

"In the scene, I was in a hotel room. I had received a text from Craig telling me what outfit I should wear. It was a black slip dress with stockings and my Manolo Blahniks. Craig came in wearing a suit, looking confident and commanding. He didn't say much, just looked at me intensely and told me what to do. He'd brought a small bag with him, and inside were...restraints and a blindfold." Tamara's cheeks flushed as she spoke, her voice growing quieter but more assured. "He tied my hands above my head to the bedpost, blindfolded me, and then just...took his time with me. I couldn't see what was coming next or control anything. All I could do was feel."

Craig's expression transformed from shock to intrigue. I could see his mind working, processing this revelation about his partner's desires.

"Tamara, that's incredibly valuable information," I responded warmly. "And Craig, how are you feeling hearing this?"

"Surprised," he admitted. "But also...intrigued." He turned to face Tamara directly. "I had no idea you wanted that. All this time, I've been trying to be gentle and considerate because I thought that's what you needed."

Tamara looked up, meeting his eyes perhaps for the first time since our session began. "I didn't know either, not really. I mean, I knew I liked those scenes in the book, but I never connected it to what might be missing in our sex life."

"This is exactly why understanding core desires is so transformative," I explained. "What we're seeing here is a perfect example of how mismatched approaches—not mismatched desires—can create sexual disconnection. Craig, you've been giving Tamara what you thought she wanted, which was tenderness and consideration. Meanwhile, Tamara, you've been craving an experience where you can surrender control and responsibility and allow Craig to be more assertive."

"But how does this work with my core desires?" Craig asked. "I want to feel wanted and desired, but in Tamara's fantasy, she's passive and I'm doing all the pursuing."

"That's a brilliant observation, Craig," I said. "And this is where the magic happens—when we look deeper at what each of your desires actually means. Tamara, when you imagine surrendering control to Craig in that hotel room scenario, how do you think that would make Craig feel?"

Tamara considered this, tilting her head thoughtfully. "Well... he'd probably feel pretty powerful. And wanted, because I'd be responding to everything he did."

"Exactly. And Craig, if Tamara was responding with genuine arousal and pleasure to your dominance—if she was moaning, arching her back, clearly lost in the sensations you were creating—how would that feel?"

Craig's eyes lit up with understanding. "I would feel powerful and in control, which I think I could do, but it's still not the same as Tamara initiating sex with me and showing me her desire."

I turned to Tamara. "Craig brings up an important point. We also have to ensure that Craig's core desires are met."

Tamara looked at Craig. "I think that if you were more controlling and dominant in the bedroom, which would definitely turn me on, I would want to have more sex with you and would initiate more frequently."

"Exactly," I told them. "When you know that your core desires are going to be met, your interest in sex increases significantly. Good sex begets more good sex."

## YOUR CORE DESIRES ARE FORMED FROM CHILDHOOD WOUNDS

To understand the origin of your core desires, you need to go back to Chapter 4 and reexamine your core childhood wounds. According to Danielle Harel and Celeste Hirschman, in your sex life, your core desires will play out in one of two ways:

1: **Resolution**. During sex, a childhood wound can be repaired by completing a missing experience. In my own life, as a child, I was responsible for meeting all the emotional needs of my narcissistic mother. I also felt totally invisible—I spent hours upon hours playing alone by myself. So, it makes perfect sense that in sex, my main core desire is to be submissive and lose control. Also, because I felt so invisible as a child, another core desire is to be completely exposed, as if to say, "Here I am. You can't ignore me anymore."

2. **Repetition with Agency:** In this version of healing a childhood wound, sex becomes the method to repeat the circumstances of the wound while maintaining control and agency which were lacking when the wound was inflicted. An example of this is a child who was heavily controlled by their parents growing up and felt like they were on a tight leash and as an adult enjoys having their partner put a leash around their neck and boss them around. This type of sexual experience, during which the now grown child maintains agency, echoes but transforms their earlier childhood experience.

I've also had clients who had been raped fantasize about or even play out having their partner or others tie them up and force themselves upon them. While reading this might make you uncomfortable, it's actually a very empowering way to heal the past trauma. To be clear, the act of rape is all about violence. Repeating this type of experience with agency is about playing in the kink world of *consensual non-consent.*

Through this process, your core desires become the balm for soothing your childhood wounds, which can be a very healthy and healing experience.

When I explained the origin of core desires to Tamara and Craig, it immediately became evident that Craig's core desires stemmed from his childhood experience of feeling overlooked by his parents, who were both high-achieving professionals consumed by their careers. As the middle child of three, Craig often felt invisible and unimportant, desperately competing for any scrap of attention or acknowledgment. His core desire to feel wanted and irresistible was clearly his psyche's attempt to heal that early wound of feeling unseen and unvalued.

"I never thought about it that way," Craig slowly said, processing this connection. "But yeah, growing up I always felt like I had to work so hard just to get noticed. My older brother was the star athlete, my younger sister was the family princess, and I was just...there."

Tamara's pattern was equally clear but represented the other healing pathway—repetition with agency. As a child, she had been raised by an extremely controlling mother who micromanaged every aspect of her life from the clothes she wore to the boys she dated.

Her mother's control felt suffocating and disempowering, leaving Tamara with little sense of autonomy or choice. Now, in her sexual desires, she was recreating that experience of being controlled—but this time, she held the ultimate power to consent, to stop, to choose when and how to surrender.

"It's strange," Tamara reflected, her voice thoughtful. "I spent so many years rebelling against my mother's control, moving across the country for college, choosing a career she disapproved of, marrying Craig partly because she thought he wasn't ambitious enough. But in the bedroom, I crave giving up control entirely."

"The difference," I explained, "is that this time, the control is consensual. You're *choosing* to surrender power to someone you trust, someone who cares about your pleasure and wellbeing. It's the opposite of your childhood experience, even though it might look similar on the surface."

## YOUR SEXUAL MOVIE: ANOTHER AVENUE TO CORE DESIRES

If you're struggling with identifying your core desires, which is all too common, especially for women who struggle with fantasies and haven't had what they would consider a peak sexual experience, there is another way to decipher them. As I discussed in *Living an Orgasmic Life*, in discussing the concept of core erotic themes, we're going to borrow a page from *Making Love Real* by Celeste Hirschman and Danielle Harel and examine what they call your "Hottest Sexual Movie."

Essentially, we all have a unique "sexual movie" that turns us on and expresses our core desires. Hirschman and Harel identify four basic themes to these movies that drive the plot, if you will. They are:

The Romantic Movie

The Passionate Movie

The Dominant/Submissive Movie

The Spiritual Movie

If you're like me, you can probably step in and play a role in any one of these movies. You might even have a favorite movie that's your biggest turn-on. But what we're looking for in this exercise is the movie that really resonates with you. Once you know that, you will be one step closer to identifying your core desires.

## *EXERCISE: IDENTIFYING YOUR HOTTEST SEXUAL MOVIE*

Examine the themes in each of these movies. Review the phrases below and notice which ones you resonate with. Make a list of all those phrases and any others that occur to you. Share with your partner how you define each of these movies (for example, what does romance mean to you, and how do you want to be romanced?) and the phrases that you would like a partner to use for each of these movies. Then practice with each other, because these phrases may feel foreign in the beginning.

***Romantic Movie:*** This movie is about being deeply cared for and loved. It contains a timeless, 'forever' quality. It is one of the most common movies in our culture, embodying the Cinderella fantasy.
*Phrases to Try*:
Timeless attraction: "You are the most beautiful woman I've ever seen."
Preciousness: "Being close to you means the world to me."
The one and only: "I've never loved someone the way I've loved you."
Physical appreciation: "You are so hot." "You smell so good."

***Passionate Movie:*** This is also one of the most common movies. It portrays intense, animalistic, insatiable desire.
*Phrases to Try:*
Tell them what you want to do to them: "I could spend hours licking and teasing you."
Share the intensity of your physical need: "I want you to be inside me right now."
Share how strongly you feel about them: "When you touch me, I get a chill running through my body and feel myself getting wet."
Talk about how much they delight you: "I love the sounds you make when you come."

***Dominant/Submissive Movie:*** This very common movie is about power. It may be that you are powerless (submissive) or that you are in control (dominant).

*Phrases to Try*

Command: "Spread your legs." "Get on all fours."

Revoke permission: "Did I tell you it was okay to look at me? Look at the ground."

Praise: "You've been a very good boy."

Punish/degrade: "You're a dirty little slut."

Disapprove: "I told you to stick your tongue inside of me. Is that as far as you can go?"

Possess: "That cock is mine! I'll tell you when you can touch it." "You belong to me, and I will do with you as I please."

***The Spiritual Movie:*** This movie can encompass multiple aspects that create a deep level of connection to oneself, others, spirit, and the universe. It includes sacred sexuality, a sense of oneness, nature-oriented connection to the elements, and the energetic blueprint.

*Phrases to Try:*

"I want to become one with you."

"I want you to bloom inside of me."

"I want to make love to you under the stars with the river roaring beside us and feel our connection to the earth."

"We must have been soulmates in a past life."

"I want to breathe you deeply into my soul."

"Let's lose ourselves completely in the void of nothingness."

Now that you have an overview of Core Desires, I do highly recommend reading *Coming Together* if you want to take a deep dive. Now let's turn to the world of fantasy.

## EMBRACE YOUR FANTASIES

Justin Lehmiller, a researcher at the Kinsey Institute and author of *Tell Me What You Want*, has penned the most comprehensive book about sexual fantasies to date. Lehmiller interviewed over four thousand adults (diverse in age, gender, sexual orientation, and background) in his landmark study.

Some of his key findings:

- Fantasies are universal, and people who regularly fantasize have more satisfying sex lives.
- Top three fantasies across the board
  - Group Sex—Having this type of fantasy was reported by 89 percent of men and 87 percent of women. This includes threesomes, orgies, and multiple partner experiences.
  - BDSM/Power Dynamics—60 percent of women and men had submission fantasies, while 78 percent of men and 55 percent of women had domination fantasies. This demonstrates that both genders enjoy the interplay of dominance and submission.
  - Romantic/Passion—92 percent of women and 83 percent of men reported romantic and passionate fantasies (including of eye contact, slow sex, and sex with love), showing that emotional connection is a common part of fantasies for both women and men.
- Novelty and Adventure is a frequent fantasy theme; some common fantasy features are having sex outdoors, or in unusual places.
- A significant number of heterosexual women (33 percent) reported same-sex fantasies.

## Fantasy vs. Reality

While knowing your fantasies can be a doorway to understanding your core desires, it's important to recognize that not all fantasies need to be acted upon. In fact, many people enjoy fantasies precisely *because* they remain in the realm of imagination. The taboo nature of some fantasies—particularly those that involve non-consent, extreme power dynamics, or experiences that would be harmful in reality, or ones that feature mythical creatures—often contributes to their arousal potential.

As Lehmiller found in his research, most people understand the difference between fantasy and reality. They may fantasize about scenarios they would never actually want to experience. This is perfectly normal and healthy.

Take Elena, a successful corporate attorney who came to me for coaching. During our sessions, she revealed that one of her recurring fantasies involved being "taken" by multiple men without her explicit consent. This fantasy troubled her deeply.

"Does this mean something's wrong with me?" she asked, her voice filled with shame. "I'm a feminist. I've built my career on empowerment and equality. How can I be turned on by something that goes against everything I believe in?"

I leaned forward, offering her a reassuring smile. "Elena, there's absolutely nothing wrong with you. What you're describing is one of the most common female fantasies. The key distinction is that in your fantasy, you maintain complete control—you're choosing to imagine this scenario, you can stop or change it at any time, and you're experiencing pleasure from it. That's entirely different from actual nonconsensual situations."

Elena's shoulders relaxed slightly. "But why do I want to fantasize about losing control when I've worked so hard to gain it in my professional life?"

"That's exactly why," I explained. "Your fantasy serves as a counterbalance to the intense responsibility and decision-making you carry every day. In your fantasy, you lose that control and unburden yourself from all your real-life responsibility."

One of my favorite resources on women's fantasies was written by actor and activist Gillian Anderson. For her 2024 book *Want*, she invited thousands of women to anonymously share their fantasies. It's a fascinating window into women's desires, which Anderson has helped to bring into mainstream culture, and I highly recommend you read it.

## But What If I Don't Have Fantasies?

This question comes up most often when I work with women. Lehmiller addressed it by recognizing that a very small percentage of individuals (just 5 percent) reported never having a sexual fantasy. Honestly, I am surprised by that statistic, given how frequently I hear this from my female clients, but they likely do not grasp that their desire to be romanced by their partner is also considered a fantasy. I also believe (and Lehmiller's research confirms this) that shame and fear of being judged are two of the biggest blocks to sexual fantasies.

If you struggle with fantasies, relax and just focus on what feels good and what you like. I often recommend that women start reading erotica and watching movies, mainstream films or female written and directed porn, and notice if there are book or movie scenes that turn them on. Start journaling about them and begin to identify the feelings that you experienced. I realize now that even during my decades of sexual dormancy, I got turned on reading and rereading Anne Rice's Vampire

Chronicles, and not surprisingly, being bitten on my neck is a huge turn-on for me. Identifying your Hottest Sexual Movie can also be a window into understanding your fantasy life. Be patient and kind to yourself and recognize that it's possible, but statistically unlikely, that you're in the 5 percent of the population who do not have access to fantasies.

I also want to acknowledge that going into fantasy in order to get yourself turned on while you are with a partner is completely normal, and you should not feel shame about this or feel like you're cheating on your partner. Your brain is your biggest sex organ, and going into your fantasy may be part of your arousal pattern. This can be particularly helpful for many individuals with low libido issues, trouble with orgasms or arousal, or erectile dysfunction.

Understanding your core desires and fantasy life is not merely an intellectual exercise—it's the foundation for creating the passionate, fulfilling sex life you crave. When Tamara and Craig left my retreat, they had a roadmap for transformation. Six months later, Craig sent me a text: "We're having the best sex of our lives. Thank you for helping us find each other again."

This transformation didn't happen overnight. It required both partners to step outside their comfort zones and communicate with unprecedented honesty. Craig had to learn to embrace his naturally dominant tendencies, while Tamara practiced expressing her desires for surrender. Most importantly, they both had to release the shame around their authentic sexual selves.

The journey to sexual authenticity requires courage. It means acknowledging that your desires may not align with societal expectations or even with your own preconceived notions about who you should be in bed. It means having conversations that feel vulnerable and scary. But in the end, it's all worth it.

# CONCLUSION

## YOUR ROADMAP TO CREATING A LIFETIME OF PASSIONATE INTIMACY

As you've just experienced, every couple has their own *Intimacy Equation*—a mix of love, desire, trust, and presence that defines their relationship. Discover yours and receive my free **Intimacy Reset Audio Practice**, a short guided experience to help you and your partner reconnect through touch and presence.

Start here with my **Intimacy Equation Quiz** https:/www.howtoimprovemylovelife.com

It is my fervent hope that this book has helped you to recognize that intimacy isn't just about sex—it's about creating emotional safety with your partner, cultivating emotional resilience, communicating vulnerably, and embracing your deepest desires. Throughout these chapters, you've also learned about all the different blocks to intimacy: unhealed emotional wounds, differences in the languages of emotional intimacy, silence, shame, and disconnection.

I'm delighted that you've read this book, and it's likely that you've experienced many flashes of recognition—moments when you truly related to a couple whose experience you've read about in this book, sharing in their frustrations and hopefully finding inspiration in their story. But actions speak much louder than words, so how do you turn this book into action so you can create a lifetime of passionate intimacy?

## THE ROADMAP: CORE PILLARS TO PRACTICE

### 1. Heal Your Wounds

As you've learned, your childhood wounds form your emotional intimacy blueprint and deeply impact your relationship with your partner. They also are the origins of your core desires, so identifying and understanding them is a core component to creating passionate intimacy. In this process, be sure to be gentle and compassionate with yourself, and seek outside help if you're feeling overwhelmed or stuck. Also remember that intimate relationships are the most potent vehicle for healing your wounds. Take this journey together, allowing both of you to discover how your individual histories shape the way you connect with each other.

## 2. Practice Emotional Intimacy Daily

I tell all the couples in my practice that five minutes a day of emotional connection will dramatically improve their relationship. Be religious about making time for a five-minute daily check-in with your partner, whether that's just eye gazing, practicing attunement, or expressing feelings using the emotions wheel. Remember that these are all skills that each of you can learn regardless of your intimacy blueprint, and that the more you engage in this type of practice, the more you will deepen your emotional intimacy.

## 3. Repair, Repair, Repair

Practice repairing conflicts using the exercises in Chapter 7. There is no question that the difference between a healthy long-term relationship and an unhealthy one is the ability to repair conflicts in a timely manner. Repair builds intimacy and trust in each other and in the relationship. I know it might seem easier to bury conflicts under the rug, but this only creates a growing mound of resentments beneath the surface, like a volcano waiting to blow.

## 4. Create Your Own New Sexual Paradigm

Talk open and freely about your sex life; share your desires, fears, and boundaries. Put a weekly sexy date on the calendar, and remember to touch your partner for your own pleasure. Learn your own and your partner's sexual styles and experiment and explore. Remember, you don't know what you don't know, and the possibilities are endless.

## 5. Embrace Your Core Desires and Fantasies

Understanding and receiving what you want to feel from sex moves sex from the bottom of the to-do list to the very top. As you explore each of your core desires, be careful to avoid judgment and shame. Remember that they emanate from your childhood wounds and help to soothe and heal them. Share your fantasies with your partner. You don't necessarily have to act them out, but even just sharing them can be a huge turn-on. Ninety-five percent of individuals have fantasies, so if you're struggling with discovering yours, give yourself time and start exploring books and films that arouse you in some way.

## 6. Stay Curious

A strong body of research validates that curiosity in all aspects of life, not just sex, leads to more long-lasting and satisfying long-term relationships. Stay curious about your own experiences and desires, as well as your partner's. Intimacy is a journey that will inevitably have some ups and downs, but as long as you stay on this path, you'll find your way to deeper connection and more passionate intimacy.

## 7. Be Patient

Transformation doesn't happen overnight. Be patient with yourself and your partner as you implement these practices. You may find that old patterns resurface, especially during times of stress or conflict. This is completely normal and is part of the growth process. What matters is your commitment to showing up authentically and doing the work, even when it feels difficult or uncomfortable. Don't be afraid to reach out for help if you're feeling stuck or overwhelmed or are experiencing high levels of distress. Sometimes it does take a village—a therapist, coach, or trusted friend who can offer perspective when you're too close in to see clearly.

I encourage you to revisit this book periodically. As your relationship grows and evolves, you'll likely discover new insights. The couple you are today is different from the couple you were when you picked up this book, and still more different from the couple you will be twelve months from now.

You now have the tools not only to repair what's broken, but to build something extraordinary—a connection where intimacy is not a byproduct of sex but is truly at the heart of your relationship. Here's to more connection, greater pleasure, and deeper intimacy!

# RESOURCES

## EMOTIONAL INTIMACY

*Hold Me Tight* by Sue Johnson. Little, Brown Spark, 2008.

- A groundbreaking guide to using attachment theory to deepen emotional bonds and strengthen love.

*The Gifts of Imperfection* by Brené Brown. Hazelden, 2010.

- Encourages vulnerability and authenticity as pathways to connection and wholehearted living.

*Making Love Real: The Intelligent Couple's Guide to Lasting Intimacy and Passion* by Dr. Danielle Harel and Celeste Hirschman, MA. Somatica Press 2015.

- A comprehensive view of emotional and sexual relationship dynamics

*The Seven Principles for Making Marriage Work* by John Gottman and Nan Silver. Harmony, 2015.

- Evidence-based insights from decades of research on what makes relationships thrive.

*Fierce Intimacy* by Terry Real. Goop Press, 2022.

- Teaches couples how to embrace conflict as an opportunity for deeper connection and truth-telling.

## SEXUAL INTIMACY

*Living an Orgasmic Life* by Xanet Pailet. Mango Publishing, 2018.

- A personal and practical guide to healing sexual trauma, awakening pleasure, and reclaiming desire.

*Come as You Are: The Surprising New Science That Will Transform Your Sex Life* by Emily Nagoski. Simon & Schuster, 2015.

- Explains the science of female sexuality and how context, stress, and self-compassion affect desire.

*Mating in Captivity: Reconciling the Erotic and the Domestic* by Esther Perel. Harper, 2006.

- Explores the paradox of desire in long-term relationships and how to sustain erotic aliveness.

*She Comes First: The Thinking Man's Guide to Pleasuring a Woman* by Ian Kerner. HarperCollins, 2004.

- A modern classic on female pleasure that redefines sexual satisfaction and mutual fulfillment.

*Coming Together: Embracing Your Core Desires for Sexual Fulfillment and Long-Term Compatibility* by Dr. Danielle Harel and Celeste Hirschman, MA. Somatica Press 2019

- • How to embrace your core desires for sexual fulfillment and long-term compatibility

*Better Sex Through Mindfulness* by Lori Brotto. Greystone Books, 2018.

- • Offers mindfulness-based practices to increase sexual desire and presence, especially for women.

## Repair & Reconnection

*Getting the Love You Want* by Harville Hendrix. St. Martin's Griffin, 2019.

- • Introduces Imago Relationship Therapy, helping couples transform conflict into connection.

*Wired for Love* by Stan Tatkin. New Harbinger, 2012.

- • Blends neuroscience and attachment theory to help couples create secure and lasting bonds.

*Eight Dates* by John Gottman and Julie Schwartz Gottman. Workman Publishing, 2019.

- • Guides couples through meaningful conversations that build trust and intimacy, and that facilitate relationship repair after conflicts.

*Attached* by Amir Levine and Rachel Heller. TarcherPerigee, 2010.
• Explains adult attachment styles and how they impact romantic relationships and repair after conflicts.
*The State of Affairs* by Esther Perel. Harper, 2017.
• Examines why people cheat and how couples can rebuild trust and intimacy after betrayal.

## Practitioners

The Somatica Institute has trained over fifteen hundred certified Somatica sex and intimacy coaches throughout the United States and the world and maintains a robust directory of recommended coaches:
https://www.somaticainstitute.com/sex-coach-near-me/

# Sexual Exploration & Kink Resources

***Application*** (available for iPhone or Android): OMGYES

For an in-depth tutorial on how to touch the clitoris, I highly recommend purchasing the OMG Yes app. Not only will you see videos of real women demonstrating different ways to touch the clitoris, but you will also be guided to practice techniques in real time on a touchscreen, using responsive animations that simulate vulvas. The app prompts you to try different strokes, pressures, rhythms, and patterns—allowing you to explore, adjust, and get immediate feedback in a safe, private way.

More information: www.omgyes.com

Purchase and download app: https://start.omgyes.com/join

***Books***

*Smart Sex: How to Boost Your Sex IQ and Own Your Pleasure* by Emily Morse. Harper-Collins, 2023.

- • A friendly, practical guide from the host of *Sex with Emily* on how to communicate desires, overcome shame, and embrace sexual confidence.

*The Erotic Blueprints: Discover Your Unique Path to Sexual Freedom* by Jaiya. Harmony, 2024.

- • Explains the five Erotic Blueprints—Energetic, Sensual, Sexual, Kinky, and Shapeshifter—and how understanding them can expand your pleasure and intimacy.

*Smart Girl's Guide to Kink* by Lee Harrington. Mystic Productions Press, 2015.

- • A clear and affirming introduction to conscious kink, boundaries, consent, and creating safe, empowering erotic experiences.

*Playing Well with Others* by Lee Harrington and Mollena Williams. Greenery Press, 2012.

- • A welcoming and humorous guide to exploring kink and BDSM communities while maintaining safety, communication, and respect.

*The Erotic Mind* by Jack Morin. Harper, 1995.

• A psychology-based exploration of how fantasy, desire, and emotion shape erotic experience and fulfillment.

*The Dominance Playbook: Ways to Play with Power in Scenes and Relationships* by Anton Fulman. Greenery Press, 2019.

- A • compassionate roadmap for those who want to explore kink together while staying connected, safe, and emotionally attuned.

## Queer Sex Resources

*Queer Sex 101: A Queer Pleasure Guide for Women and their Lovers* by Allison Moon (with KD Diamond). Lunatic Ink, 2015.

- An inclusive, illustrated guide to queer women's sexuality that blends practical how-to advice with humor, personal stories, and a celebration of pleasure and consent.

*Ask a Queer Chick: A Guide to Sex, Love, and Life for Girls who Dig Girls* by Lindsay King-Miller. Plume, 2016.

- A witty, down-to-earth, advice book offering honest guidance on love, sex, identity, and queer community from a proudly lesbian perspective.

*The Joy of Gay Sex* by Charles Silverstein and Edmund White. HarperCollins, 1992 (revised editions).

- A pioneering and sex-positive classic that combines explicit instruction, emotional insight, and cultural context to celebrate intimacy and pleasure between men.

# ACKNOWLEDGMENTS

This book would not have been written had it not been for guidance from some of my spiritual mentors, Patricia Barrett and Ziba Wood, two beautiful, kind, and compassionate guides who have supported me through the last six years as I've built my Passionate Intimacy Retreat business. Both individually and collectively, they have seen me through challenges with my health, business, and relationship. In many of our sessions, they both were able to see something I could not. Despite my protestations, there was indeed another book inside of me. For their love and unwavering support, I am most grateful.

My dear friend and brilliant colleague Kai Wu was instrumental in helping me fine-tune the final version of this book. Kai opened my eyes to some blind spots and helped ensure that the book was inclusive of straight and queer people. Her words of encouragement kept me going as I struggled to cross the finish line. I'm also deeply grateful for the contributions of Leslie Doares, an awesome couples therapist who has been on this journey with me for a decade; she is part of my wonderful Mastermind group of Bad Ass Bitches, and we recently celebrated our tenth anniversary.

Huge thanks to Brenda Knight and her amazing team at Books That Save Lives. She continues to believe in me and the power of the written word to transform lives, and I am extraordinarily grateful that she included me and this book in her new publishing company.

Last but certainly not least, I am forever grateful for Daren Love, the literal love of my life, who has put up with my crazy hours, my ADHD, and my mood swings over these past six months. His support and love have held me through this process and have allowed me to explore my deepest edges and experience the passionate sex and intimacy I've craved my entire life.

# APPENDIX: EXERCISES

The following exercises are designed to help you and your partner integrate the practices from *The Intimacy and Repair Kit* into your daily life, deepening emotional connection, trust, and passion over time.

# REFERENCES


Bourbeau, Lise. *Heal Your Wounds and Find Your True Self*. Éditions E.T.C., 2000.

Brizendine, Louann. *The Female Brain*. Morgan Road Books, 2006.

Brown, Brene. *Daring Greatly: How the Courage to be Vulnerable Transforms the Way we Live, Love, Parent and Lead*. Avery, 2015.

Chapman, Gary. *The 5 Love Languages: The Secret to Love That Lasts*. Northfield Publishing, 1992.

Fern, Jessica. *Polysecure: Attachment, Trauma and Consensual Nonmonogamy*. Thornapple Press, 2020.

Glickman, Charlie, and Emirzian, Aislinn. *The Ultimate Guide to Prostate Pleasure*. Cleis Press, 2013.

Harel, Danielle, and Celeste Hirschman. *Coming Together: Embracing Your Core Desires for Sexual Fulfillment and Long-Term Compatibility*. Somatica Press, 2019.

Harel, Danielle, and Celeste Hirschman. *Making Love Real: The Intelligent Couple's Guide to Lasting Intimacy and Passion*. Somatica Press, 2015.

Jaiya. *Your Blueprint for Pleasure*. Harmony, 2023.

Kerner, Ian. *Passionista: The Empowered Woman's Guide to Pleasuring A Man*. HarperCollins, 2008.

Lehmiller, Justin. *Tell Me What You Want: The Science of Sexual Desire and How It Can Help You Improve Your Sex Life*. Da Capo Lifelong Books, 2018.

Martin, Betty. *The Wheel of Consent: The Art of Giving and Receiving*. Betty Martin, 2017.

Morin, Jack. *The Erotic Mind: Unlocking the Inner Sources of Passion and Fulfillment*. HarperCollins, 1995.

Nagoski, Emily. *Come as You Are: The Surprising New Science That Will Transform Your Sex Life*. Simon & Schuster, 2015.

Pailet, Xanet. *Living an Orgasmic Life: Heal Yourself and Awaken Your Pleasure*. Mango Publishing, 2018.

Schnarch, David. *Passionate Marriage: Keeping Love and Intimacy Alive in Committed Relationships*. W.W. Norton & Company, 1997.

Somatica Institute. *9 Steps to Successful Relationship Repair*. Somatica Institute, 2022.

Winston, Sheri. *Women's Anatomy of Arousal: Secret Maps to Buried Pleasure*. Intimate Arts Center Press, 2010.

https://www.psychologytoday.com/us/blog/the-myths-of-sex/202309/how-common-are-sexless-marriages?utm_source=chatgpt.com

https://www.sexandpsychology.com/wp-content/uploads/Kinsey-Report_Updated-Cover.pdf

https://www.somaticainstitute.com/blog/9-steps-to-successful-relationship-repair/

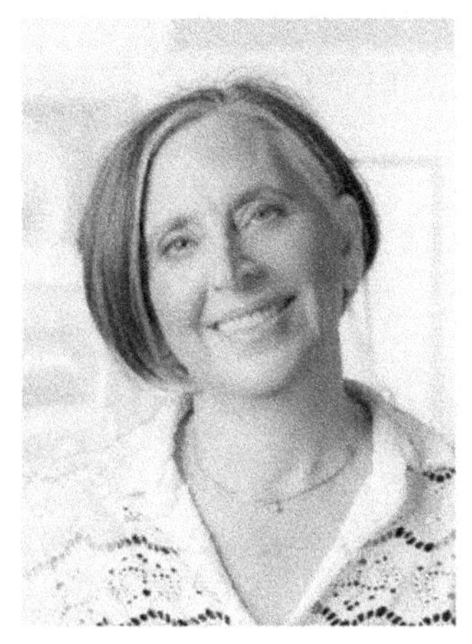

Xanet Pailet is the best selling author of *Living an Orgasmic Life: Heal Yourself and Awaken Your Pleasure (2018)* and *The Sex & Intimacy Repair Kit: How to Enhance Communication and Create a Lifetime of Passionate Intimacy (2026)*. She is the founder of Passionate Intimacy Retreats where she has led over 100 couples' intimacy retreats. Xanet is a former NYC health care lawyer who lived in a sexless marriage for over two decades. At age 50, after experiencing her own sexual healing and awakening in 2011, she transitioned her career into a full-time sex and intimacy educator and coach and trauma practitioner.

Xanet believes that pleasure is our birthright and she is passionate about helping individuals find their way back into their bodies, their desires, and their pleasure. Over the past decade, she has helped rescue hundreds of couples from unsatisfying sex lives and has helped women who are sexually shut down learn how to love themselves, their body, and reclaim their desire.

Xanet is a certified Somatica Sex and Intimacy Coach, Sexological Body Worker, Holistic Pelvic Care Practitioner, Tantra Educator and Somatic Experiencing Trauma practitioner. She has been on the faculty of 1440 Multiversity, Ecstatic Living Institute and the Somatica Institute. Connect with Xanet at passionateintimacyretreats.com.


instagram.com/xanetpop

facebook.com/xanetpop

linkedin.com/in/xanet-pailet-2b464671

youtube.com/@thepowerofpleasure8132

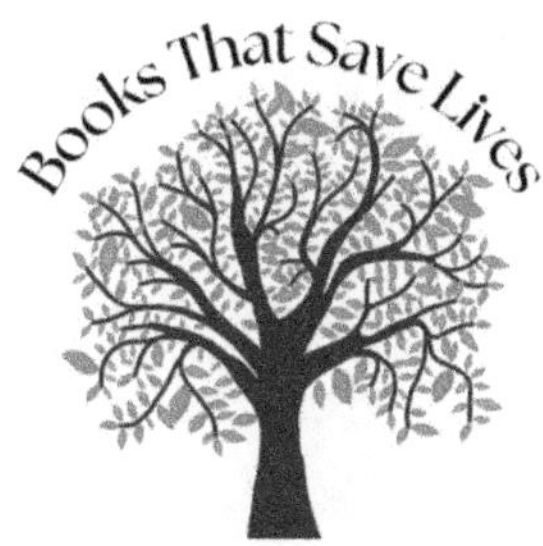


Books That Save Lives came into being in 2024 when the editor and publisher, Brenda Knight, heard directly from readers and authors that certain self-help, grief, psychology books, and journals were providing a lifeline for folks. We live in a stressful world where it is increasingly difficult not to feel overwhelmed, worried, depressed, and downright scared. We intend to offer support for the vulnerable, including people struggling with mental wellness and physical illness as well as people of color, queer and trans adults and teens, immigrants and anyone who needs encouragement and inspiration.

From first responders, military veterans, and retirees to LGBTQ+ teens and to those experiencing the shock of bereavement and loss, our books have saved lives. To us, there is no higher calling.

We would love to hear from you! Our readers are our most important resource; we value your input, suggestions, and ideas.

Please stay in touch with us and follow us at:

www.booksthatsavelives.net

Instagram: @booksthatsavelives

www.ingramcontent.com/pod-product-compliance
Lightning Source LLC
Chambersburg PA
CBHW032052090426
42744CB00005B/187

* 9 7 8 1 9 6 3 6 6 7 4 1 7 *